YOUR 6 WEEK PLAN

Sarah Turner and Lucy Rocca

Published by Accent Press Ltd – 2013

ISBN 9781783752058

Printed and bound by CPI Group (UK) Ltd, Croydon, CR0 4YY

THE SOBER REVOLUTION: YOUR 6 WEEK PLAN

Time Please, Ladies!

By Lucy Rocca

All of us experience sparks of ideas in fleeting moments; a sudden decision to live another way or to enact a deep and lasting change to the person we are inside. Frequently these monumental thoughts disappear into the ether before we have time to grab on to them and set about putting them into practice. The classic example is those we experience at the end of a particularly wonderful holiday during which we have lived differently to the norm and want desperately to maintain that new way of living once we arrive back home.

And then something happens or rather, things happen; the kids need help with their homework and/or taking to football practice or a horse riding lesson, the fridge is empty and the house needs a damn good clean, the dog has just run in from the garden and left muddy footprints all over the newly-polished wooden floor demanding it be mopped for the third time in a day, and the ironing pile is almost touching the ceiling ... and those little gems that sparked so briefly quietly dissipate, forgotten and lost to the mountain of unrealised dreams in the back of our minds.

So how can you take hold of a desire to change, put it into practice and live your life differently on a permanent basis? For me, the notion that I would one day eradicate alcohol from my life built up gradually over a five year period. There was no sudden flash of lightning that by itself served to provide me with the tools I needed to become alcohol-free – in contrast I experienced several events during my early thirties that accumulated and eventually became a great big, no arguments, refusal isn't an option, one-way ticket to booze-free living. I took it with both hands.

The final push that saw me transformed from a reckless, irresponsible person who lived for wine and nights out, to a calm, happy, contented, and self-assured woman, happened when I woke up in hospital after a particularly heavy night of alcohol bingeing. I perceived this to be some kind of warning, fully acknowledging that I wouldn't always be so lucky as to be discovered (unconscious and vomiting on a deserted pavement late at night) and taken to A&E by a friend if I were to continue drinking myself into such oblivion. But the capacity to commit to an alcohol-free life was pretty much already present, that night's events merely providing the last piece of the jigsaw that, once complete, would see me waving goodbye to the Wine Witch for good.

For many people, however, taking the final step to cutting alcohol out of their life for good does not emerge as the result of such a frightening incident as being rushed to hospital, passed-out drunk and scraping the bottom of the barrel. For the vast majority, becoming alcohol-free is a lifestyle option that is borne out of an accumulation of growing fed-up with being hungover, regularly losing control to the point of acting in an embarrassing manner, piling the pounds on and feeling lethargic, anxious, and suffering from low-level depression. And because there is no wham moment where we know absolutely, categorically, forever that we need to stop what we're doing, sticking to a sober lifestyle can easily fall by the wayside just as soon as the last regrettable drunken occasion has been forgotten.

Just as is often the way when embarking on a new diet (you know the scenario; shortly before departing on holiday you nip to town to purchase a bikini, pick one out that is perhaps slightly optimistic in terms of sizing and as you stare at the bulging flesh in the changing room mirror, the tiny pants digging into your muffin top and two boobs magically becoming four under the strain of the minuscule cups, you declare 'That's it! I'm going on a diet!'), the moment of inspiration is incredibly forceful and real, only to waft away into a distant memory a few hours/days later when a cake presents itself before you, impossible to resist.

So exactly how can you ensure that a very real wish to extract yourself from the grip of an alcohol dependency (most likely

2

bobbing back up to the surface of your thoughts following yet another embarrassing/shameful/hangover-inducing booze fest) can be transformed into a long lasting action plan to live (happily) alcohol-free?

Getting firmly into the land of alcohol-free living (and ensuring that you stay there without the Wine Witch luring you back into destructive old habits) requires a degree of forward planning. Knowing what emotions to expect once the old crutch has been kicked away, preparing for the potential pitfalls and learning how to work through cravings will all stand you in good stead when it comes to maintaining your alcohol-free lifestyle. Developing an alcohol dependency is very similar to getting involved with a thoroughly unsuitable partner. Your relationship began with excitement and passion but eventually dwindled into a tedious cycle of pleasure-seeking swiftly followed by a blanket of regret. We do not always recognise that someone is having a destructive effect on us at the start of a new relationship, and when we eventually realise this it can be extremely difficult to end things because we have grown emotionally dependent upon them. As for booze, that first glass is the longed-for rendezvous with Mr Unsuitable, after a day spent bogged down with the humdrum of domesticity and/or work. But we need to recognise the negative and destructive consequences that this relationship is having on our lives and find the courage to finally give Mr Unsuitable the boot.

Becoming sober and learning how to be happy with regards to your decision to live without booze amounts to so much more than merely pouring all the remaining wine in the house down the sink – living as a non-drinker takes some getting used to, especially if the drinking has been protracted and heavy. Maintaining an alcohol-free approach means finding out who you really are beneath the falsity of booze and learning how to interact socially without your old alcoholic prop. It means experiencing raw emotion and discovering how to cope with negative situations without drinking the problem away.

Quitting alcohol can lead to uncomfortable truths coming to the fore; a relationship may not be all it appeared to be when under the influence of booze, underlying mental health issues such as depression or bi-polar disorder could suddenly become exposed having previously been disguised by the mood-altering effects of alcohol, and the emotions of guilt and shame arising as a result of erstwhile drunken behaviour may now demand attention, no longer so easily hidden with a constant stream of wine (or whatever's your poison). It is these wrinkles and creases which will need ironing out in the first few weeks and/or months of alcohol-free life. Ignoring deeper issues could result in the apple-cart of sobriety being upturned.

A whimsical notion of stopping drinking can quite easily never come to fruition, prevented from developing into something more concrete by not giving sufficient thought to how one might explain such a bold and (for many) radical lifestyle choice to friends and family. It's important to discover something that you will enjoy drinking as an acceptable alternative to alcohol, and a way to fill the sudden vast increase in spare time each evening. Without forward-planning, an initial rush of enthusiasm for a commitment to alcohol-free living can be quashed in no time at all, purely as a result of the individual in question not putting into place a viable plan of action and instead attempting to coast along exactly as before only minus the glass of something to hand.

Becoming a non-drinker is a completely different process for everyone and despite there being common themes (for instance what might constitute a trigger point or act as a craving eliminator), we all became heavy drinkers for different reasons, and it is these we must address if we're to have a good chance at committing to booze-free living. A lack of self-esteem and confidence in social situations is a frequently-cited reason for drinking excessively, as is struggling to cope with a bereavement or single parenthood or the breakdown of a long-term relationship; whatever the root cause, it is this which a) must be identified and b) needs to be dealt with through an alternative coping strategy other than alcohol.

4

In addition to the plethora of reasons why we as individuals come to develop our own unique dependencies upon booze, it is also worth acknowledging that Western culture (in which we are all submerged) holds alcohol in high esteem and is one which promotes it ubiquitously. Should you be one of the many who finds herself unwittingly dependent on this addictive substance, then to extricate yourself from its tenacious grip can be incredibly challenging when all around us are messages of how alcohol injects our lives with glamour, sophistication and fun.

As further reinforcement to the alcohol industry's campaign of promulgating alcohol as an essential social lubricator and utterly acceptable feature of most people's lives, there exists in society a very negative perception of those who choose to be non-drinkers. Because those who have freed themselves from this marketing trap are in the minority, this way of life which should be considered normal is in actuality regarded by many as being odd, and that by not partaking in regular binge drinking a person is weird and anti-social. This social pressure is another reason why remaining AF can sometimes prove to be an uphill struggle.

So just how should one go about the task of cutting alcohol out of one's life for good? Because the reasons for abusing alcohol and the level of dependency differ from drinker to drinker, a useful approach to becoming AF is to create a personalised plan of action.

Consider the initial phase of your new completely AF life as the beginning of a road of self-discovery – cutting alcohol out of your life is all about being honest with yourself and learning who you truly are beneath the alcoholic fog. Becoming AF requires huge amounts of inner strength, soul-searching and determination; the best way to beat the Wine Witch is to ensure that you have all the ammunition (right from the start) required for sober success.

'The Sober Revolution; Your 6 Week Plan' is a journal in which to log your own personal experience of becoming alcohol-free. As anyone who has ever attempted to stop drinking permanently only to fall off the wagon a few weeks down the line will know, after sufficient time has lapsed the rose-tinted glasses can appear and magically wash away all the bad memories of our drinking days, replacing the negatives with a glittering spectacle of all that can be found at the bottom of a bottle. By logging your journey from booze slave to happy, liberated, and AF, you can record exactly how alcohol made you feel on the last occasion you drank to excess, establish the reasons behind your destructive relationship with booze and work out a pragmatic approach to beginning life afresh, free from the alcohol prison.

As you embark on this new alcohol-free stage of life it is important to ascertain exactly what you would like to do differently now; are you looking for increased self-esteem, weight loss, a sense of being in control of your own destiny, or eradication of the weighty burden of guilt and regret, both of which have built up over the years as a direct result of too much booze? Are you hoping to be a better parent, with increased patience and understanding, or to earn back the respect of those around you who have grown weary of your drunken antics?

Whatever the driving force behind your decision to live alcohol-free, it is a great idea to record why you have made this choice and to chart your progress as the days become weeks and you begin to see the results you were hoping for. It is difficult to recognise any substantial changes in ourselves as they occur so gradually; by logging your thoughts and achievements you can create a permanent reminder of exactly why sober living works for you, and why it is preferable to your old existence of drinking, hangovers, mood swings, lack of productivity and shame.

I often regard my approach to becoming alcohol-free for good in the early phase as being akin to going into battle – just possessing a vague desire to quit boozing is not going to withstand the force of years and years of mental hard-wiring, weighty social pressures, and the alcohol industry's clever marketing techniques that are often so effective in presenting alcohol as totally innocuous, sophisticated, and civilised. In order to beat the Wine Witch, you need ammo.

Unearthing the techniques that work best for you is, once again, a personal matter. For me, nothing blasts my stress away more efficiently than a good long run with the dog, iPod on loud as I pound the pavements and clear my head, but that is for many people their idea of hell. Whenever I become aware of those old feelings of sinking into a quagmire of negativity that always used to lead to full-blown depression with vats of vino thrown into the mix, I meditate, or take the dog out to the Peak District, or have a long soak in the bath with candles burning and a face mask on – I have learnt how to take care of myself in a kind and helpful way, and those are my tools for remaining alcohol-free.

Alcohol consumption when engaged in to excess takes up large chunks of a drinker's life, and those empty hours will need to be filled with something once the last of the booze has been poured down the sink. Take some time in the early weeks to experiment with a variety of activities until you happen upon the ones you really enjoy – members of Soberistas partake in knitting, yoga, running, or cycling to name just a few, but what works for one won't necessarily work for another. Open your mind and set out to have some fun with whatever hobby you choose to road test; the end goal is to find a pastime that you can really get stuck into, something you can build on and enjoy long-term.

Without wishing to pull out the scare tactics, it is also worth reminding yourself of the many and serious health implications of sustained and heavy consumption of alcohol. Fatty liver is a common ailment/disease found in alcohol-dependent people and up to 15% of those who continue to drink will develop cirrhosis within ten years. A study of risk factors for early-onset dementia placed alcohol misuse at the top of the list (in contrast, the influence of hereditary factors is small, according to research in this area).

Three times more alcohol is now consumed per head as in the 1950s and it is estimated to cause 30,000 to 40,000 deaths a year. In addition to bowel cancer and breast cancer, there is also evidence that alcohol increases the risk of cancers of the liver, oesophagus, mouth, pharynx, and larynx. In total, scientists estimate alcohol causes 20,000 cases of cancer a year.

Of particular interest may be the fact that women who regularly drink three glasses of wine a night increase their risk of developing breast cancer by a whopping 50%. Breast cancer has soared in recent decades, with new cases doubling since the early 1970s. In part, this has been driven by the rise in alcohol consumption. It is now the most common cancer, with almost 49,000 cases and 12,000 deaths a year.

In knocking booze on the head, you are not only empowering yourself and providing your mind and body with a far greater shot at a happy and fulfilling life, but you are instantly reducing the risk factor in all of the above health implications (and many more – alcohol is the known culprit behind sixty different medical conditions).

If you have read *The Sober Revolution* then you'll already be armed with the background as to why we believe alcohol is best left alone, and just how amazing life can be once the booze blinkers have been removed. By creating 'Your 6 Week Plan' you can now put the theory into practice and develop your own personal armoury for keeping the Wine Witch at bay, and placing you firmly in the happy land of alcohol-free living.

At the back of Your 6 Week Plan you'll find the Compendium – this section of the book is filled with ideas for recipes (food and drink) that will help you in your endeavours to stay AF, and a variety of other useful snippets for you to dip into as you work your way through the coming weeks.

Best of luck on your sober journey!

Lucy and Sarah

xx

Food For Thought – Am I Really an Alcoholic?

Where would you position yourself along the following line of various drinking behaviours: non-drinker, social drinker, party animal, lush, or raging alcoholic? And what exactly is an alcoholic anyway? There is no definitive line that, once crossed, separates the apparently harmless 'life and soul of the party' from the sad alkie who has nothing but a park bench and a supersized bottle of cider to look forward to. You can't buy a test from Boots that highlights the precise moment when you move into the territory of 'problem drinking' after years of simply 'enjoying a drink.'

Speaking from personal experience, there are many people who, despite their own habit of knocking back way too much wine on a frequent basis, will view you with a certain degree of pity and concern just as soon as the truth is outed that you have chosen to become a non-drinker. It is a phenomenon that reminds me of the Hans Christian Andersen story, *The Emperor's New Clothes*. In that tale, nobody dares reveal to the Emperor that they cannot see his new and allegedly stunning garments and, rather than risk standing out as idiots, his ministers and the townsfolk all nod along with one another and agree that their leader looks fine and dandy. Nobody tells him that he is in actual fact, naked, for fear of reproach.

Once you decide to go down the alcohol-free (AF) road, you may encounter reactions from people who cannot see past the end of their own wine glass sufficiently to recognise that they too might have a 'drink problem.' Rather than acknowledge that it might not be a great idea to go out on a Saturday night and down eight pints, or drink a bottle of wine every night in front of the TV, some drinkers will transfer their concern to you (the non-drinker who is getting her life sorted out) while they persistently refuse to examine their own relationship with alcohol. There is a widespread denial going on when it comes to the issue of how much we drink in western societies.

A substantial factor behind this type of reaction is the societal perception of what an 'alcoholic' really is. For many years prior

9

to my acknowledgement of my own unhealthy relationship with booze, I (along with the majority of people in the western world, as far as I can tell) held a very particular notion as to what an alcoholic was. In my mind, one of the key defining characteristics of a person suffering from this affliction was simply that they weren't like me. I also imagined that the reasons leading to (as well as the frequency and quantity of) their abuse of alcohol, were nothing like the motivations behind my own heavy drinking. It was always very easy to find someone with a more serious problem than mine, thus letting myself off the hook for what was, essentially, a major alcohol dependency.

Here are some of the reasons that I used during my drinking days to bolster my belief that I was not alcohol dependent;

- I drank to have fun and to let my hair down but, crucially, when I actively chose to (an alcoholic was completely at the mercy of the bottle, with no self-control, merely a pathetic need to obliterate themselves that resulted in the wheels gradually, and totally, falling off).

- My own drinking was above board because I bought the bottles of wine from Waitrose, and not from a bargain basement booze store filled with cheap and nasty super-strength cider and lager.

- My habit of becoming so drunk that I passed out on the settee a couple of nights a week, or of falling over in the street virtually every time I went out drinking, was because I was having a good night out and letting my hair down (rather than bingeing on an addictive substance over which I obviously had no control).

Looking back, I recognise that there **was never any choice involved at all** – the drink had got its teeth into me a long time before I knocked it on the head.

I drank alongside teachers and nurses, lawyers, businesswomen, and businessmen. The establishments in which I socialised were, largely, expensive restaurants and sophisticated wine bars, and when I stayed at home to drink I cooked fancy meals and poured high-end wines into pretty glasses from John Lewis. This was all a million miles away from swigging out of a 2-litre bottle of 8% lager on a street corner, wasn't it? Surely none of this made me an alcoholic?

Drinking alcohol is so culturally normalised that when you do finally step outside of the booze bubble, ditch the beer goggles, and adopt the level of clarity that comes only with being a non-drinker, you become aware of the vast degree to which the world around you has comfortably nurtured your growing alcohol dependency without you even realising that trouble was brewing (excuse the pun). What also makes the decision that you have possibly overstepped the invisible line into 'problem drinking' very difficult is that there will most likely be a large number of friends and family all around you who are also 'problem drinkers', but who are firmly ensconced in the land of the Emperor's New Clothes – 'let's all pretend it's OK to get half-cut every night, and then nobody will stick her head above the parapet and actually question this behaviour.'

If you say it out loud, then you are an alcoholic; if you remain in denial and continue to drink, then you're not.

So, how to determine whether you do, truly, have a problematic relationship with the bottle? If you have got this far into reading *Your 6 Week Plan* then the chances are you are well aware that you've already stepped foot into the realm of alcohol dependency, to a degree. You may be a long way off pouring vodka over your cornflakes first thing in the morning, but that's the best place to be at when embarking on this plan. Arresting the development of alcohol addiction before the wheels fall off completely is a far better idea than waiting until the sorry end, when the stereotypical park bench alcoholic clutching a bottle of super-strength cider concealed inside a brown paper bag, is no longer such a leap of the imagination.

Alcohol is a drug, and a widely and cleverly marketed one at that, with few restrictions imposed on how, where, and when it is advertised. It is extraordinarily easy to slip into an unhealthy relationship with booze, and not even to realise it. Despite occasional concerns that may crop up with regards to the negative impact alcohol is having on one's health or family or work life, it is all too simple to persuade one's self that drinking more than government guidelines is not so bad after all (and simultaneously be carried along in the tide of public opinion).

All of this confusion and hypocrisy, in conjunction with a pervasive trend of denial when it comes to alcohol consumption, really does not help the individual who feels worried about her own personal relationship with booze.

The drive, however, to resolve problematic drinking patterns can only come from YOU. Ultimately, it is about personal responsibility and that is why we called this book *Your* 6 *Week Plan*, as opposed to *The* 6 Week Plan, or *Our* 6 Week Plan. At this point (at the very beginning of your journey to resolving your difficulties pertaining to alcohol), focus on your individual perception of alcohol. How does drinking make YOU feel? What do YOU hope might be different in your life if alcohol were no longer a part of it? What are the negatives resulting from your alcohol consumption? Have these always been a consequence of drinking or has something changed recently which in turn has affected your relationship with booze?

Forget society at large, disregard whether you are 'an alcoholic' or not. Right now, at this moment in time, it's about YOU attempting to disentangle yourself from the grip of the Wine Witch, however tenacious that grip may be. Your 6 Week Plan will help you to analyse the patterns and reasons behind your alcohol consumption, as well as providing you with tools and strategies for moving forward. If you believe yourself to have set foot on the slippery slope of alcohol dependency and, crucially, you know that you would like to get away from the danger zone and back into a place which affords you increased control over your life, health, and happiness, then it is irrelevant whether you should be labelled 'an alcoholic' or not.

For some, defining themselves as an alcoholic is the first step to recovery. Personally, I would never have described myself as an alcoholic, and still don't consider that I ever fell into that category. Yes, I relied on alcohol as a prop in all sorts of social situations, and I abused booze as a way of coping (or at least I believed it to be a coping strategy at the time) with challenging periods in my life. I also perennially lacked the elusive 'off switch' which is something I believe I will never possess. Do any of the above characterise me as an alcoholic?

Is this a question which demands an answer if one is to be truly able to deal with their alcohol-related problems and move on in life, free from addiction?

We Only Get One Life

Rather than focusing on what has been and gone, switch the whole business around in your head and direct your thoughts to the future. Make it less about being 'an alcoholic' (a label which can be impossible to shake and one which is loaded with connotations of illness, recovery, and potential 'relapses') and more about becoming a Soberista. We get one life – where is the sense in dragging around the heavy and frequently shameful burden of being 'an alcoholic' when, alternatively, we can wear with pride the label of Soberista? A Soberista is an empowered and liberated individual who has made an incredibly positive choice to cut alcohol out of her life in order to maximise her chances of enjoying health and happiness on a long-term basis.

Self-esteem and confidence, so commonly eroded with sustained alcohol abuse, are far more likely to be restored if one chooses the route of empowerment, personal responsibility and pride. #

Positive Mental Attitude

Before you begin your six week plan, have a read through the following section which will help prepare you for success – although one size never fits all, these little tips can help everyone.

13

Stay in the present tense for the first few days – avoid thinking about being AF in the long-term. Strategies and plans for this can be put into action a little further down the line.

Join soberistas.com so you can make friends with like-minded people who will know exactly how you're feeling and will be able to give you advice and support. There's usually someone around in their chat room 24/7 so you can have help whenever you need it.

Buy some supplies: One of the main things that causes your alcohol cravings is low blood sugar, so make sure you have something sweet in the house to combat this. Try dried fruit and nuts rather than sweets or chocolate, as these can play havoc with the body's chemistry and actually increase your cravings. Also, load the fridge with some of your favourite alcohol-free drinks such as ginger beer, elderflower cordial, or fruit juice, just so that you have something alternative and pleasant to reach for when your cravings do start. There are other suggestions for AF drinks at the end of the Compendium section.

Cravings only last ten minutes so make sure you have something to distract yourself with. Buy a new book or film that you've wanted for ages, or perhaps some luxurious bath products for a really relaxing bath. As you'll be saving a lot of money by cutting out the booze, you should be able to give yourself a treat. If you really need to focus your mind, use an egg timer to see how long you've got left – you'll probably have forgotten that you even wanted a drink by the time it goes off!

Get clever with money. Although your health is paramount, finances play a large part in all our lives. Organise your AF spreadsheet right now to enable you to see clearly how much you are saving by cutting out alcohol. Treat this as an investment, not just for your mind and body but for your future security too. With tangible results to enjoy, you will be further reinforcing why life is definitely better without the Wine Witch.

Cultivate some new hobbies. You'll find you have loads of free time now that you've decided to be AF – try something that keeps your hands busy but doesn't require too much thinking – knitting, cooking, or perhaps even going for walks are all great for this.

Take a picture of yourself before you start on your six week plan. Even giving up alcohol for a short period of time has major observable benefits to your body – you might be surprised at the end of the six weeks just how much weight you've lost, and how much better your skin looks now that you've beaten the Wine Witch.

Reassess your life in general. Sometimes this can be a less-than-desirable process, but unless you get honest about your life now, you risk falling into the same trap over and over again. And remember, each time you begin the process again, there is even more baggage to deal with than the last time.

Use the rating system throughout this book. You'll see it on every day of the plan. It is a good way to chart your progress as you work through the six weeks. The colour scheme works in the following way:

- **Bad**– you are struggling. Cravings are running high and emotions are all over the place.

- **Neutral** – you're keeping your head above water. Definitely room for improvement but the Wine Witch is being kept firmly in her place.

- **Good** – you're flying high. This is where you're aiming to be as much as possible. Positivity abounds!

Week 1

Week 1

Day 1

Today I chose not to drink ☐

Use the rating system below to track your mood. It will be an excellent reference to look back on! Always be honest, make notes to understand what the three ratings mean to you.

Good ☐ _____
_____

Neutral ☐ _____
_____

Bad ☐ _____
_____

This is it, the first day of the rest of your life! How do you feel? Euphoric and optimistic about your new AF life, or weighed down with dread and anxiety over how you'll cope without your old crutch? Note down your feelings below, and make sure you keep a record of all your trigger points as they occur throughout the day; to be forewarned is to be forearmed!

"And you? When will you begin that long journey into your-self?"

— Rumi

Week 1
Day 2

Today I chose not to drink ☐

Use the rating system below to track your mood. It will be an excellent reference to look back on! Always be honest, make notes to understand what the three ratings mean to you.

Good ☐ _____
_____

Neutral ☐ _____
_____

Bad ☐ _____
_____

Old habits take time to erase from your mental hard-wiring – if your cravings are getting the better of you, remember the old favourite; H.A.L.T. Never be Hungry, Angry, Lonely, or Tired. It can be very difficult to achieve all four, but busy yourself with forward planning to give yourself the best chance of success! Book in a few social occasions with friends that are staged well away from the temptations of alcohol – try the cinema, a lunchtime date, or a walk in the countryside in order to avoid loneliness and boredom. Get plenty of rest and get the fridge stocked up!

Now dig deep and write below 10 reasons why you have embarked on Your 6 Week Plan –why have you fallen out of love with alcohol? What are the worst things that have happened as a result of your drinking too much? Don't sugar-coat the truth; you'll need this page if complacency sets in a few weeks down the line …

The Soberistas Tip of the Day:
'My tip to those starting out would be to only think in bite-size chunks of time (for me, committing to a whole day was overwhelming to start with but 5 minutes I could do) – concentrate on just a few minutes in which you choose not to drink. Before you know it, those little chunks have added up to the whole evening, its bedtime and you're AF.'

Week 1
Day 3

Today I chose not to drink ☐

Use the rating system below to track your mood. It will be an excellent reference to look back on! Always be honest, make notes to understand what the three ratings mean to you.

Good ☐ _____

Neutral ☐ _____

Bad ☐ _____

It is possible that you are enjoying the buzz of your new AF existence – it can be such a refreshing experience to wake up and NOT be filled with regret, self-loathing, and misery! You are well on your way now, so why not celebrate with a delicious Virgin Piña Colada?

Serves 2 (but you may want to drink it all yourself)

Ingredients

1 can cream of coconut (not coconut milk)

1 can pineapple slices plus juice

Crushed ice

In a blender, combine the pineapple juice and cream of coconut. Pour into glasses half filled with crushed ice. Put a slice of pineapple on rim of each glass and pin a cherry on the pineapple slice with toothpick if you are feeling particularly fancy. Sit back and imagine you are on a desert island – this is the most amazing drink ...

Write about what you've achieved today below:

Week 1

Day 4

Today I chose not to drink ☐

Use the rating system below to track your mood. It will be an excellent reference to look back on! Always be honest, make notes to understand what the three ratings mean to you.

Good ☐ _____

Neutral ☐ _____

Bad ☐ _____

You may be having difficulty sleeping – night times could be interspersed with sweats, unsettling alcohol-filled dreams in which you imagine you've had a drink, and endless hours spent staring at the ceiling unable to switch off. Keep a good stack of books at your bedside and plough your way through them instead of overthinking in the dark. Don't forget to write down how you feel at this stage – dig deep and unburden yourself on paper!

"Until you make the unconscious conscious, it will direct your life and you will call it fate."

— Carl Jung

Week 1

Day 5

Today I chose not to drink ☐

Use the rating system below to track your mood. It will be an excellent reference to look back on! Always be honest, make notes to understand what the three ratings mean to you.

Good ☐ _____
_____

Neutral ☐ _____
_____

Bad ☐ _____
_____

Your thoughts will no doubt increase massively during these early AF days – drinking alcohol on a regular basis results in a mental fog, its addictive nature firing up so much longing for the next drink that there is little room for any particularly productive thinking. Now that the booze has been banished, your mind will come alive again. This can be difficult to deal with at first and it may seem as though quiet headspace will for ever remain out of reach. However, things will settle down eventually and in the meantime why not consider yoga or meditation as a way of instilling some inner peace? Write about these thoughts and how you overcame them today.

The Soberistas Tip of the Day:
'The most valuable thing I employed in avoiding alcoholic abuse was to have a very distinct vision of where my life was going. One may call it 'destiny.' I envisioned my health, fitness levels, interests, body shape, sharpness of mind, and most importantly, fulfilling all of my potential. In doing this, there simply was no room for the negative effects of alcohol. I suppose I created a situation where my destiny was of such great value that alcohol became its enemy.'

Week 1
Day 6

Today I chose not to drink ☐

Use the rating system below to track your mood. It will be an excellent reference to look back on! Always be honest, make notes to understand what the three ratings mean to you.

Good ☐ _____
_____

Neutral ☐ _____
_____

Bad ☐ _____
_____

This week should be a time of retreat so make a real effort to avoid placing yourself in any tempting situations; social events where alcohol is present and readily available should take a back seat, and meal times should be adjusted in order to ward off cravings (and the meals themselves – for instance, if pasta dishes usually trigger a major red wine urge then omit such meals from your diet for a while). It's only a few days of frustration and not a lifetime of despair – tomorrow is your one-week anniversary so hang in there!

Make a list of these tempting situations so you know what to avoid:

Week 1
Day 7

Today I chose not to drink ☐

Use the rating system below to track your mood. It will be an excellent reference to look back on! Always be honest, make notes to understand what the three ratings mean to you.

Good ☐ _____

Neutral ☐ _____

Bad ☐ _____

Congratulations! You have just completed the first week of your new life! Have you noticed any improvements yet? Have friends or family let you know of any benefits they've noticed in the new AF you? If so, write them down below – try to get into the habit of rewarding yourself and being self-complimentary for your accomplishments as you build them up. Heavy drinking and self-loathing go hand in hand, but now you can begin to work on your self-esteem and being kind to yourself for a change.

Work out how much you've saved this week by not drinking alcohol and go and treat yourself – yes, you really do deserve it!

"One reason I don't drink is that I want to know when I am having a good time."

–Nancy Astor

Lucy's Blog – Reasons Why I Drank, August 24th 2012

I started drinking heavily in my mid-teens and continued to do so until I hit 35. I often think about the factors that led me to drink alcoholically, because I know it was more than simply sustained exposure; right from the off I drank to get drunk, and I never, ever got it when people professed to sipping a glass of wine 'with dinner,' or to 'blowing the froth off a couple' on the way home from work. When I poured the first glass of the night, it was with one intention in mind; to down as much booze as I could get away with before I either a) passed out or b) ran out of alcohol, whichever came first.

People often said to me that I was lacking some kind of inherent 'off switch,' a magic voice that I consistently saw manifest itself in others, and for which I craved longingly, a voice that would tell me to stop when I had had enough; a watchful guardian in my head, telling me to go home while I could still stand.

I have always been a funny bugger, in that I am most definitely an introverted extrovert, or an extroverted introvert, or some such contradiction. Shy on the outside with a lot going on inside and an obstacle sandwiched between the two, preventing the voice inside from being heard. Reason number one why I drank – I am actually a little bit shy, and often struggle to have conversations with people who I don't know very well. Thus the discovery of the following equation was (for a long while) the key to social success: shy girl + wine = chatty and fun girl. Over time, the equation morphed in to this: shy girl + wine = annoying idiot.

Early on in my teens I developed a rabid interest in the opposite sex. I don't recall ever being struck with a debilitating shyness around boys, but I do know that once I threw some alcohol in to the mix, the dating game became a whole lot easier. So, reason number two; being sexy and intoxicating to the male of the species becomes easy as pie when you have knocked back a bottle of wine. Ditto the above; over time, shy girl + wine = annoying idiot of a girlfriend.

I get bored very easily. I often feel as though life is just slipping through my fingers like sand, and I am overwhelmed by a desire to make it all 'the cream.' I don't do banal very well. Alcohol injects fun (for me, this is really an illusion – I recognise that now. When I drank, I thought that those brilliant nights when everyone lets their hair down and bonds over meaningless conversations, and quiet nights at home transform after a few bottles have been drunk to dancing in the living room, I thought that somehow they were real. Like Primal Scream said, 'we are together, we are unified').

But I wasn't unified and together with anyone; I was becoming discombobulated. On many nights I would find myself waking up in the early hours in a strange bed in the dark, in someone's spare room, where someone had carried me because I had got drunk and embarrassing. Until the penny dropped, there was reason number three: get drunk and life gets more fun. Reason number four was to drown out the darkness, to forget my worries. Number five, to mask loneliness. And number six, the most stupid of all, to sufficiently wipe away the self-hatred and shame that coursed through every inch of me, owing to the vast amount of alcohol I had consumed the night before.

And the truth is that every feeling that I tried to suppress, every social interaction that I tried to lubricate, and every personality trait that I tried to fake, has blown away like a puff of smoke, now that the glass is empty. Whatever you try to escape from through drinking, it will still be there in the morning.

Sarah's Blog – Dealing with the Fear, March 5th 2013

For most of us, to say that we are apprehensive about our decision to become AF is an understatement. Without alcohol many of us are nervous and shy, which plays a large part in our love affair with booze. Perhaps some of us have a fear of life in general. Drinking allowed us to be outrageous on occasion, as well as giving our confidence a boost.

Inevitably, if you have looked for help you have also realised that liberation is now a problem. This is always progressive, and much further down the line the fear becomes whether or not you can make it until booze o'clock, or even past lunchtime without a snifter. That creates the fear of being found out, or embarrassing yourself or loved ones.

The fear now, however, might be more to do with not ever being able to drink again, which can seem a prospect almost too difficult to bear. There is so much fear it almost swallows you up.

Sobriety means dealing with fear in a different way. You have to re-wire. One of the best phrases to help with this is **that courage is fear in action**. Inaction leads to fear. It very soon becomes clear that thinking about what could happen (and we usually imagine the worst case scenario) is far worse than what actually happens.

So now imagine the outcome of not drinking, rather than the build-up to it. Think about the fear – or, even better, talk about it. This is a very intimate subject, and we tend to beat ourselves up over any perceived weakness. It's vital to try to eradicate this, as only then will your confidence grow. Since you stopped drinking, there may have been no inappropriate outcomes. You might have failed to put a point across, but hopefully you have not been ashamed, guilt-ridden, or embarrassed. At the height of our intoxication there was no fear, so getting to grips with new coping mechanisms is another part of your job and is really important for your emotional wellbeing.

So there is real benefit from being proactive. Try to never allow the void created by *not* drinking become unused and wasted. This can be a very satisfying part of the journey, and can show us how much simpler, and more positive, life is without alcohol.

Week 2

Week 2
Day 1

Today I chose not to drink ☐

Use the rating system below to track your mood. It will be an excellent reference to look back on! Always be honest, make notes to understand what the three ratings mean to you.

Good ☐ _____
_____

Neutral ☐ _____
_____

Bad ☐ _____
_____

Have you noticed how much longer the evenings seem now that you've knocked the booze into touch? Have you given any thought to how you're going to fill your time? Learning to prioritise yourself amidst the whirlwind-busy lives that many of us lead is vital – try your hand at a few pastimes over the coming weeks and when you find something you like, stick at it, and always make time for it each day.

A few suggestions – board games, crochet, baking, sewing, learning a foreign language, or how to play a musical instrument, gardening, writing poetry, painting, photography, rock-climbing, knitting, yoga, joining a gym, swimming, hiking … the list is endless. Make a list of a few of your ideas:

The Soberistas Tip of the Day: 'My tip would be to really take it slowly and give yourself some YOU time. In life we don't spend enough time on ourselves which results in us getting stressed. By taking some time every day to live in the moment really helps me. Whether it is running, crochet, or just sitting like I am now with my glass of tonic! It is when I don't do this that I end up with the occasional wobble! So ME TIME is my number one tip!'

Week 2
Day 2

Today I chose not to drink ☐

Use the rating system below to track your mood. It will be an excellent reference to look back on! Always be honest, make notes to understand what the three ratings mean to you.

Good ☐ _____

Neutral ☐ _____

Bad ☐ _____

This is the week you start to get honest with yourself and everyone you care about. The secrets and lies have to go – like de-cluttering your wardrobe, this is the start of clearing out your headspace. As you work through this period of emotional turbulence you may suffer extreme mood swings – perhaps consider warning your nearest and dearest and ask for a little extra patience. Don't forget to keep writing your feelings down – use the space below as a confidante during those moments when nobody else seems to understand.

Week 2
Day 3

Today I chose not to drink ☐

Use the rating system below to track your mood. It will be an excellent reference to look back on! Always be honest, make notes to understand what the three ratings mean to you.

Good ☐ _____
_____

Neutral ☐ _____
_____

Bad ☐ _____
_____

Rather than continuing to wear the booze aisle blinkers, now's the time to begin experimenting with alternatives – avoid restricting your choice to either water or fruit juice. There are some gorgeous AF drinks out there so get taste-testing! The ritual of drinking is all part of the booze trap, so establish a new ceremony around quaffing your favourite AF drink. Don't fall into the easy habit of denying yourself special drinks simply because you no longer choose to drink alcohol. Conjure up a different and delicious mocktail each evening as a reward for your fantastic decision to live AF!

Why not get in touch with your inner child and whip up a milkshake? Try this one for starters!

Banana & Honey Milkshake

Ingredients

1 Banana

1 dollop of honey (try Manuka honey and benefit from its immunity-boosting properties too!)

1 glass of milk

2 scoops of vanilla ice cream

Combine all these in a blender and blend for a scrumptious milkshake.

Don't forget to address your feelings below:

Lucy's Blog – Things (not) to do in Barcelona, August 22nd 2012

As a result of eating fewer cakes, drinking fewer lattes, and going for more runs, I have lost a total of about five pounds in as many weeks. Seems like a lot of sacrifice for a small reward, but at least the number is going in the right direction, and I am no longer dreading standing on the scales as I did in the final trimester of pregnancy. My weight during those last few months was increasing by about three or four pounds a week – I did wonder where it would end. Thankfully, I am fairly confident that I can wear my new (humongous on the chest coverage, due to breastfeeding boobs which resemble watermelons) bikini on the beach, without being fearful that Greenpeace might get called to drag me back in to the water.

So we leave in four days for Mallorca; I have bought my miniature toiletries, new suitcase, and aforementioned monstrous bikini. The dog is booked in for kennels, the British summertime is winding down and it looks like we will fly out of Manchester amidst pouring rain and chilly temperatures – always pleasing when you will depart at the other end of the flight straight in to thirty-five degrees and glorious sunshine.

And this holiday will, of course, be sans booze. There was a time when I couldn't imagine going away and not drinking, when I would almost not have seen the point of a holiday if it didn't include alcohol. And there were many holidays when booze was consumed on a nightly basis and good times were had by all, the wine adding to the general merriment and relaxed evenings that everyone wants from their week in the sun. But in the last few years there were many times when I drank not to be sociable and fun and relaxed, but to get hammered; when I drank alcoholically.

Example; Barcelona, the Ramblas, circa 2004. My travel companion and I hit the beers mid-afternoon, and continued to sink many cerveza de pequeñas in thirty-five degree heat (not really relevant – if it had been minus ten, we would still have got as wasted as we did. I'm using the temperature as a bit of

44

an excuse here) well into the night. My memory is a little cloudy but I remember sitting in a plaza, people-watching, and downing my third or fourth drink. Time then becomes fluid; snippets of conversations flicker through my mind but vast gaps emerge leaving me with a staccato recollection of the latter part of the evening.

An argument sprang up between us (there is a theme here, me + boyfriend + alcohol = massive fight) which led to two members of La Policia intervening in what they thought was a domestic violence matter (I was acting like a melodramatic idiot, and my boyfriend was holding on to me while he attempted to calm me down; this was construed as him assaulting me). After a lengthy altercation between the four of us in downtown Barcelona, we were allowed to leave and scarpered back to our hotel, him muttering about my inability to hold my drink, me blaming him for attracting the attention of the police. It was messy, embarrassing. We fell in to liquor-induced comas upon reaching our hotel bedroom, approximately three hours before we had to be up for the journey home.

Plane departure time; 0800 hours. Time we awoke; 0700 hours. Panic. We grabbed the clothes that were strewn around the room, bundled them in to our cases, and ran downstairs to check out. Somewhere amidst the previous evening's activities, the strap across the top of my Birkenstock sandal had come unstuck, leaving me with a shoe-shaped piece of cork and a flap of white leather as one half of my footwear. In my hungover state of mind this troubled me, so much so that as we raced through Barcelona airport with minus five minutes before take-off, I discarded the sad-looking sandals in to a rubbish bin and veered in to a shoe shop in order to purchase a more respectable-looking pair. Oh, the joy on my boyfriend's face! Boarding the plane fifteen minutes post-departure time, we received the obligatory round of applause that passengers award to the crap, hungover people who almost miss their flight due to over-refreshing themselves the previous evening.

This holiday will be sans booze, sans drunken arguments,

sans broken sandals. There will be no fracas with the local constabulary, no almost-missed flights. There will, however, be relaxing afternoons spent by the pool, bowlfuls of patatas bravas, our baby's first swim, browsing in dark, Mallorcan shops for souvenirs, and a photo album's worth of happy holiday pictures for my family to return to time and time again. I can't wait.

Week 2
Day 4

Today I chose not to drink ☐

Use the rating system below to track your mood. It will be an excellent reference to look back on! Always be honest, make notes to understand what the three ratings mean to you.

Good ☐ _____
_____

Neutral ☐ _____
_____

Bad ☐ _____
_____

By now the reality of the entire sobriety subject could be sinking in and there may also be The Fear to contend with; the fear that your plan to live AF might actually work, and also that you might never *want* to drink again. It can be a frightening prospect to deal with life in the raw. You may already have experienced a few tricky life situations since having your last drink which you have had to cope with stone cold sober for the first time in a long while. How did you manage?

However scary things may seem now, don't panic! You're doing great, and as time goes by these instances will only get easier to handle, as you become better acquainted with your inner self.

"You don't need to drink to get over your feelings. Deal with your feelings – that's how you get over them."

— Holly Hood, *Prison of Paradise*

Week 2
Day 5

Today I chose not to drink ☐

Use the rating system below to track your mood. It will be an excellent reference to look back on! Always be honest, make notes to understand what the three ratings mean to you.

Good   ☐   _____
                                   _____

Neutral   ☐   _____
                                   _____

Bad   ☐   _____
                                   _____

Are you sleeping OK? By the end of this week sleep should be less problematic. What will be less welcome is the probable tiredness that may dog you throughout the day. Remember that you are no longer filling up on rocket fuel, or feeling the effects of the adrenaline that pumped around your body caused by the shame, guilt, and the worry that you might be breathalysed at 7.45 a.m.

Focus on developing a bedtime routine – a luxurious and pampering bath followed by a hot, milky drink and a good book in bed usually works wonders. Or if you're feeling decadent, why not treat yourself to a new silky nightdress and a manicure in bed? Write some ideas below, and why not add this Ginger Ale Bellini to them while you're at it?*Serves 1 (it's all yours!)*

Ingredients

1 ripe peach, peeled and diced

Ginger ale

100 g sugar

150 ml water

In a small pan, dissolve the sugar in the water over a low heat (do not boil) to make a syrup. Blend the peach in a blender and mix in enough of the syrup to sweeten to taste. In a fancy, tall glass, pour in the ginger ale to approximately the halfway point. Add the peach puree slowly and stir carefully, ensuring the liquid only reaches ¾ of the glass. Top up with a little more ginger ale. And relax ...

Week 2
Day 6

Today I chose not to drink ☐

Use the rating system below to track your mood. It will be an excellent reference to look back on! Always be honest, make notes to understand what the three ratings mean to you.

Good ☐ _____
_____

Neutral ☐ _____
_____

Bad ☐ _____
_____

You may be feeling as though it's been forever since you last gave into the Wine Witch but don't let down your guard just yet – it's still early days and depending on how long you have been regularly drinking, your brain will take a fairly substantial length of time to fully rewire itself.

Have you read any books about becoming AF? Remind yourself that you are engaged in a mental battle which could last a few weeks or even months yet – arm yourself with as much ammo as possible; reading books about moving on from an alcohol dependency is a brilliant way to speed up the process of reconfiguring your neurological pathways. Brainwash yourself!

Write about a victory that you achieved in your mental battle today:

The Soberistas Tip of the Day:

'I buy expensive chocolates, cordials, coconut water, and an array of beautiful magazines to fill the treat-shaped hole. Oh, and I drink from elegant glasses.'

Week 2
Day 7

Today I chose not to drink ☐

Use the rating system below to track your mood. It will be an excellent reference to look back on! Always be honest, make notes to understand what the three ratings mean to you.

Good ☐ _____
_____

Neutral ☐ _____
_____

Bad ☐ _____
_____

Hurray – you have now been sober for two whole weeks! Have you noticed any physical signs yet that your body is enjoying this new healthy and happy way of life? Maybe you've lost a bit of weight, your skin might be looking less dull and your eyes have perhaps begun to sparkle once again.

With the money you've saved over the last week by not drinking alcohol, buy yourself a gorgeous treat. Yes, you truly deserve it!

"'Could I have a Sloe Gin Fizz, without the gin?'

'What's the point of that, Miss?' the waiter said.

'Tomorrow morning.'"

— Libba Bray, *The Diviners*

Week 3

Week 3

Day 1

Today I chose not to drink ☐

Use the rating system below to track your mood. It will be an excellent reference to look back on! Always be honest, make notes to understand what the three ratings mean to you.

Good ☐ _____
_____

Neutral ☐ _____
_____

Bad ☐ _____
_____

Physically you should by now be feeling considerably better – if not, there's no need to worry; we are not all the same, and it's never how you start that counts. You are detoxing, it takes time, and we are all unique. For many people, this is the stage when complacency can set in; the first couple of weeks are often plain sailing, but now is the time when the thought may arise – 'Did I actually have a problem in the first place?'

If this thought has been plaguing you, try **Playing the Movie to the End**. We all have a picture in our heads of the first drink. This is the picture we drink on – glamorous, refreshing, relaxing, and harmless. In our minds, the image sticks there and we never play the film through to the end. Now is the time to get into the habit of doing exactly that – work your way through the sequence of events until you reach the final frame. For some it will be a total car crash, for others it will be very sad and lonely. You know where it will end. This is a helpful, but sometimes painful, trick.

Write down a brief description of how your own booze movie plays out here (and no censorship!):

Lucy's Blog – I Choose, February 26th 2013

When I stopped drinking alcohol I acknowledge that I spent a few weeks, if not months, in recovery. By this I mean that I invested a fair bit of energy in dealing with a newly discovered concept – emotions. Previously, I had poured vast amounts of Pinot Grigio or Chardonnay down my throat whenever I split up with a boyfriend, was not successful in a job interview/promotion, got rained on, received a large and unexpected bill, graduated, had a birthday, received some surprising and happy news, and so on ... basically, I was not accustomed to listening to my feelings and subsequently I was not familiar with acting upon them in a positive and helpful way.

It wasn't particularly pleasant at times, all that 'getting to know myself' stuff, and there were many occasions when I felt like throwing the towel in, marching up the road to my local and getting stuck into a nice bottle of their finest dry white and a packet of 20 Marlboro Lights. But I didn't.

A little voice inside, quiet but impossible to ignore, told me that if I gave in now I would be undoing all of my good work and propelling myself back to square one, where I would have to begin the whole sorry business of 'recovery' once again. And so I persevered.

After several months I stopped experiencing any negative thoughts about living alcohol-free and instead, adopted a thoroughly different mind-set; one which made me see that I am, in fact, a chooser – and being someone who has the freedom to choose a lifestyle that is so positive and good for the soul is an empowering and wonderful thing. At that point, I ceased to regard myself as being 'in recovery' and realised that I was RECOVERED and could now get on with the business of living.

I will always be a person who cannot simply have 'one for the road' or 'a sneaky after-work pint' – for me alcohol was, and for ever will be, an all-or-nothing substance. But I most certainly do not consider that this makes me an alcoholic forever, or in recovery forever – not at all. I made a choice to stop drinking, and I continue to practice that choice every day because I am A CHOOSER. This is what I choose: I choose to wake up energised and with no regrets every morning.

I choose to be the best parent I can be without ever jeopardising my children's safety or emotional security.

I choose to invest all my time and energy into worthwhile people, projects and activities.

I choose to maintain a good level of health and physical fitness, thus optimising my chances of not dying prematurely of cancer, liver failure, or heart disease.

I choose to spend my money on things that I need and which add value to my life or to that of my family.

I choose to not poison my body with toxins and mind-altering substances that depress my central nervous system, making me anxious and prone to dark moods, or make me say or do things which will fill me with shame and self-hatred. I choose to not spend hours of each week agonising over whether or not I can have a drink of alcohol or not.

I choose to get to know myself, free of any external and false influences – I give myself the chance to be me. I choose to give myself the best possible chance at happiness.

Week 3

Day 2

Today I chose not to drink ☐

Use the rating system below to track your mood. It will be an excellent reference to look back on! Always be honest, make notes to understand what the three ratings mean to you.

Good   ☐   _____
                       _____

Neutral   ☐   _____
                       _____

Bad   ☐   _____
                       _____

Questions are probably being asked about why you are no longer drinking, but remember – you are not answerable to anyone except yourself and loved ones, so just keep it simple and comfortable. Write down a few potential 'answers' here to help you feel prepared if someone does give you a grilling about why you are now a non-drinker: _For example – 'I don't have a reliable "off switch" and I got fed up of always drinking more than I intended.'_

Week 3

Day 3

Today I chose not to drink ☐

Use the rating system below to track your mood. It will be an excellent reference to look back on! Always be honest, make notes to understand what the three ratings mean to you.

Good ☐ _____
_____

Neutral ☐ _____
_____

Bad ☐ _____
_____

If you are not skipping along in a pink cloud of euphoria with regards to your new sober life, take a few minutes now to examine the areas of your life that have shown a marked improvement since you sank your last glass. You most definitely should be functioning better in general, and the alcohol-fuelled chaos that can be so disconcerting should have dissipated. That said, you may still be asking yourself, 'What's the point if I can't have a drink?' This can always be countered by reminding yourself that there was never much point in spending time and money on beautiful new outfits and afternoons in the beauty salon only to go out and get wasted, rendering you unable to remember anything at all of your big night out. You are a goddess-in-waiting; focus on all the plus points – remember, there was nothing very glamorous about passing out drunk on a regular basis!

Write below 10 improvements to your life since you became AF:

The Soberistas Tip of the Day:
'For me the uppermost thought in my mind for every day is acceptance; accepting that I have the problem first of all, but also accepting the fact that we can't change anything else but ourselves and our own behaviours. Along the way we come across so many obstacles and difficult people and situations that we can do absolutely nothing about ... it's life, it happens. We have to accept it for what it is and do the best possible job we can do for ourselves. That and gratitude for all the many good things that are going on around us if we only take the time to look.'

When I first emerged from the wreck that my alcohol dependency had created, I felt battered and small – my personality had been manipulated and shaped by addiction and shame for so long that I no longer knew who I was. I'm not sure if, in the first few weeks, I truly believed that I would never drink again. There was an element of self-doubt that teased my newly sober self with the thought that I couldn't do it, that over time I would forget the horror of my last encounter with booze and I would cave in and begin to drink again. But I chose to stop drinking for a sufficiently long enough period to allow myself the first taste of being me without the prop of alcohol, and during that time I recognised and learnt things about myself and my relationship with booze that cemented my commitment to teetotalism. A major step forward was to admit to myself that I had a dependency upon alcohol.

The UK Alcoholics Anonymous website states that while they do not offer a formal definition of alcoholism, the majority of their members would agree on the following statement: "... it could be described as a physical compulsion, coupled with a mental obsession. What we mean is that we had a distinct physical desire to consume alcohol beyond our capacity to control it, in defiance of all rules of common sense. We not only had an abnormal craving for alcohol but we frequently yielded to it at the worst possible times. We did not know when (or how) to stop drinking. Often we did not seem to have sense enough to know when not to begin."

This description fits perfectly with my relationship with alcohol, but it took several weeks of being sober for me to recognise that I was an alcohol addict. As soon as I took a sip from my first drink, my mind would begin to whir frenetically, as it attempted to map out the most effective way to consume as much booze as possible before someone intervened and told me I had had too much. This was the reason why drinking alone was always so much more enjoyable for me – there was never a killjoy leaping forward to impose their own restrictive behaviour upon me, when all I wanted to do was get hammered.

And so, armed with this newfound awareness, I slowly accepted that I was dependent upon alcohol and therefore I had a responsibility to those around me, and to myself, to stop for good. No single factor would have been sufficient in prompting me to get on top of my problematic relationship with booze – rather, elements in my life began to come together like a jigsaw puzzle that, once complete, presented something of a eureka moment to me.

The years of destructive and shameful behaviour and the associated self-hatred, age, and a growing sense of mortality that grew at the same rate as my youthful ignorance of personal responsibility diminished, meeting my fiancé and developing an awareness of who I really was without the façade of drinking – it was all of these things that pushed me in to that place where I had wanted and needed to get for so many years. And now, here I am – nineteen months of sobriety and what feels like a lifetime of self-discovery later, a much calmer, honest, more confident woman who is enjoying a normal existence after twenty-one years of self-abuse.

I knew that I had come on leaps and bounds when on holiday last week, as I didn't miss alcohol one bit; conversely, if someone had put a bottle of Pinot in front of me and told me that I could drink it with none of the associated negativity, without the hangover or the guilt or the damage to my health, I would have happily walked away.

Week 3
Day 4

Today I chose not to drink ☐

Use the rating system below to track your mood. It will be an excellent reference to look back on! Always be honest, make notes to understand what the three ratings mean to you.

Good ☐ _____
_____

Neutral ☐ _____
_____

Bad ☐ _____
_____

Enough time has passed since your last drink to allow you time to reflect on all the negative repercussions of your alcohol consumption. Try not to sink into a pit of despair and regret – while it's important to recognise how badly booze impacted on your life and those who are close to you, now is the time to work on boosting your self-esteem. Concentrate more on all the positives of being AF, less on the gloomy consequences of your alcohol-fuelled history.

Write down 3 fabulous personal characteristics that have emerged as a result of you becoming AF:

"It takes courage ... to endure the sharp pains of self-discovery rather than choose to take the dull pain of unconsciousness that would last the rest of our lives."

— Marianne Williamson, *Return to Love: Reflections on the Principles of 'A Course in Miracles'*

Week 3
Day 5

Today I chose not to drink ☐

Use the rating system below to track your mood. It will be an excellent reference to look back on! Always be honest, make notes to understand what the three ratings mean to you.

Good ☐ _____
_____

Neutral ☐ _____
_____

Bad ☐ _____
_____

Have you noticed a few pounds being shaved off the weekly grocery shop? Drinking an average-priced bottle of wine a night, plus a few extra over the weekend, adds up to approximately £50 – £60 per week. Throw in the little extras associated with a boozy lifestyle (taxis, cigarettes, maybe late-night pizza when you get the munchies) and you might be looking at saving around £5,200 every year by becoming AF! Write down some ideas for what to do with your savings, and next time you go shopping, pick up a watermelon, a couple of limes, a packet of fresh mint, and some coarse sea salt, and treat yourself to a Watermelon

Margarita:

Ingredients

1 watermelon

Four cups of ice cubes

2 limes (or more if you prefer)

Coarse sea salt

Sugar

De-seed a watermelon and slice the flesh up into inch-thick slices. Then put the watermelon flesh into a blender with four cups of ice cubes.

Juice the limes, and add the juice coarse sea salt, and sugar to taste (this is a matter of personal preference so experiment a bit and write down your chosen amounts. I use the juice of two limes and a good pinch of both the salt and sugar).

Blend the mixture until smooth and totally free of lumps. Pour into a jug and garnish with sprigs of mint and wedges of lime (and a couple of cocktail umbrellas if you are feeling fancy!)

Sit back and enjoy!

Lucy's Blog – Out with the Negative, in with the Happy!
February 20th 2013

As a child I perpetually lived in the moment. I was lucky enough to have a very happy childhood, one that was full of Enid Blyton-esque adventures in sunny fields with friends, roller-skating up and down the cul-de-sac that I grew up on, baking cakes and biscuits, reading and writing voraciously, and never seemingly worrying about anything, past or present. I just was.

During the years that I spent drinking heavily (aged 15–35) my state of being was at a polar opposite of those younger halcyon years. Anxiety levels were astronomical, with worries over relationships, divorce settlements, my daughter's wellbeing, how much I was drinking, paying the bills, whether I was causing my body untold harm through all those cigarettes and bottles of wine … my mind seemed to be set to a constant whirring mode, churning and cogitating and over-thinking all these troubles that, in the end, were what they were; none of the excess pondering made the slightest indent on any of it. The outcomes were the same regardless.

Nowadays I experience 'normal' worries. A small amount of worrying does us good and if we existed in a blissful childhood state, skipping about without a care in the world, we would find our little lives running to a standstill fairly quickly. Normal worrying helps us keep a rein on our budget, encourage our children to work a little harder on their homework when they begin to spend too much time on Facebook, and put a bit more effort into our relationships if we feel they are not as tight as they perhaps might be.

A huge difference that I have noticed in the few weeks since I began to practice the art of meditation is that I seem to be able to better control those uncontrollable fits of anxiety, the ones that render you feeling sick and with palpitations: a bit like the way I felt yesterday morning on my way to the ITV studio to appear on *Daybreak*. I caught myself becoming overwhelmed with fear in the back of the car as we saw the London Eye looming out of the

72

early dawn with its blue-lit cars suspended over the Thames, my stomach churning and my mind rattling along at a hundred miles an hour. Then I made a decision to not feel that way.

Hang on a minute! It's my mind, I call the shots. I took some deep breaths, focussed my mind and cleared my thoughts. I began to consider that this experience was something to be savoured – it's not every day that you get to go on live TV and sit next to Dr Hilary! I recalled how this would have been dealt with by me as a child – I would have seen the whole journey through eyes wild with excitement, from arriving in London late at night, staying in a nice hotel, being picked up by a car with tinted windows and taken to ITV's studios … I would have loved every minute 30 years ago. Instead, I had been allowing my out-of-control worrying to ruin the whole event.

Practising meditation has allowed me to be much more aware of negative thinking patterns and has also taught me that I don't have to accept them – I can decide whether I perceive something in a positive way or a negative way. Yesterday I chose to see things positively, and I found myself enjoying the whole experience; by simply altering the way I decide to process external situations, I have also made myself a little bit braver and next time (if there is a next time) I will approach things in a far more relaxed fashion, right from the off.

Only you can determine whether you tackle things positively or negatively – taking the former option makes life a million times easier and more enjoyable!

Week 3
Day 6

Today I chose not to drink ☐

Use the rating system below to track your mood. It will be an excellent reference to look back on! Always be honest, make notes to understand what the three ratings mean to you.

Good ☐ _____

Neutral ☐ _____

Bad ☐ _____

How's your mood? If you are feeling down it may be worth a visit to your GP – regular alcohol abuse plays havoc with a person's mental state and can often disguise a plethora of underlying disorders. For those taking anti-depressants, they are used in an effort to lift a low mood but are subsequently negated by the consumption of too much alcohol – in becoming AF you may now notice your anti-depressants are working properly and the dose may need adjusting.

If you are in any doubt about your mental state, seek advice from your doctor now – underlying mental issues such as anxiety, depression, post-natal depression, and bi-polar disorder are regularly overlooked and sufferers often self-medicate with alcohol, thus exacerbating their condition. In ditching alcohol you are giving yourself the chance for a much more emotionally settled future, so now is as good a time as any to attempt to put right any unresolved problems which, if ignored, could propel you back towards the Wine Witch a few weeks down the line.

"And the day came when the risk to remain tight in the bud was more painful than the risk it took to blossom."

— Anais Nin

Week 3

Day 7

Today I chose not to drink ☐

Use the rating system below to track your mood. It will be an excellent reference to look back on! Always be honest, make notes to understand what the three ratings mean to you.

Good ☐ _____
_____

Neutral ☐ _____
_____

Bad ☐ _____
_____

You are exactly halfway through your six week plan. Where do you stand on alcohol now? Do you miss it? Has your life changed for the better or for the worse as a result of not drinking? Look back to the first day of your plan – how did you feel then? Have you altered your views on living AF since you began? If so, have you changed your feelings for better or worse?

Three weeks is a substantial length of time and you should have noticed the cravings have dwindled somewhat. You still have a long way to go, however, before the longstanding habitual thought processes related to alcohol consumption will be rewired fully. Be patient, and remember to reward yourself today; you've clocked up another 7 days of saving approximately £6 - £10 per day by not drinking. Do the math! That's between £42 and £70 to spend on a gorgeous treat – enjoy!

Week 4

Week 4

Day 1

Today I chose not to drink ☐

Use the rating system below to track your mood. It will be an excellent reference to look back on! Always be honest, make notes to understand what the three ratings mean to you.

Good ☐ _____
_____

Neutral ☐ _____
_____

Bad ☐ _____
_____

Boredom might have started to rear its ugly head if you've been avoiding social situations for fear of boozy temptation – this can be a very big danger. Hopefully you have not been beating a temperance drum and therefore there is no reason for you not to go out. You haven't got a contagious disease, and neither are you going to preach to anyone who drinks a lot.

It might just surprise you how other people really will not give a damn whether you drink or not. Just take the whole process in baby steps and have a test run or two. Real life cannot be avoided forever. Try to have at least one person on side to support you in your endeavours to remain AF. Up until now you could have used the designated driver excuse but there has to come a point where you need no excuse at all not to drink; it's simply a choice you have made about how to live your life.

Write below how you feel with regards to socialising minus your old prop:

Your loved ones should slowly be starting to rebuild their trust in you. Gone are the days when you tried desperately to avoid them all so you could start your drinking in peace.

Week 4
Day 2

Today I chose not to drink ☐

Use the rating system below to track your mood. It will be an excellent reference to look back on! Always be honest, make notes to understand what the three ratings mean to you.

Good ☐ _____
_____

Neutral ☐ _____
_____

Bad ☐ _____
_____

Are you a people-pleaser? This can often be driven by guilt and it needs to be addressed at this stage. 'No' is a difficult word for many women, and when you were caught up in the dreadful trap of low self-esteem and zero confidence as a result of alcohol abuse you more than likely said 'yes' when you didn't really mean it, purely in an effort to make amends for your drinking behaviours. Try very hard to get out of that habit – you know your own mind now, so start being honest with both yourself and those around you.

Can you think of 3 instances when you said 'Yes' recently when you really wanted to say 'No?' Write them down here, along with the reasons why you felt you couldn't be honest. Think about what the outcome may have been had you said 'No' instead.

Week 4

Day 3

Today I chose not to drink ☐

Use the rating system below to track your mood. It will be an excellent reference to look back on! Always be honest, make notes to understand what the three ratings mean to you.

Good ☐ _____
_____

Neutral ☐ _____
_____

Bad ☐ _____
_____

You should by now be noticing an increase in mental clarity. Hopefully those days of old when you simply muddled through with a fuzzy head operating at half speed are now a distant memory.

How have you been spending your evenings? Perhaps you'll have begun to notice how much more spare time you have now that you are AF – plus you'll be able to remember all the good times you are having as opposed to waking up with patchy memories of the night before and a cold feeling of dread in the pit of your stomach. Still looking for something to fill your evenings? Don't be scared to dip your toe into waters unknown; this is a time of self-discovery, your own little adventure, so have a whirl, do something a bit different. Who knows where it will take you?

Use this space to jot down a few ideas of those things you've always fancied having a go at …

The Soberistas Tip of the Day:

'The best tip has to be joining Soberistas.com as it's available 24/7. Being able to remain anonymous has allowed me to be completely honest for the first time about my relationship with alcohol, and has been so liberating for me. I love the solidarity, friendship, support, shared experiences, encouragement, and understanding which was so unexpected. I feel quite determined not to blip as it would feel to me like wasting all the support from everyone here who has so helped me be strong.'

Week 4

Day 4

Today I chose not to drink ☐

Use the rating system below to track your mood. It will be an excellent reference to look back on! Always be honest, make notes to understand what the three ratings mean to you.

Good ☐ _____

Neutral ☐ _____

Bad ☐ _____

Have you dropped a few pounds since cutting out alcohol? Booze is laden with empty calories – a large glass of wine (250 ml) contains around 230 calories, the same as a Cornetto ice cream! If you were regularly downing a bottle a night, you were drinking the calorific equivalent of a Big Mac and a small portion of fries! As long as you haven't been filling the booze gap with loads of supersize bars of chocolate then you should have witnessed a loosening of your jeans.

Weight management becomes a MUCH easier business when you remove alcohol from the equation. Have you noticed any positive physical changes that have come from becoming AF?

"We cannot direct the wind but we can adjust the sails."

— Author Unknown

Week 4

Day 5

Today I chose not to drink ☐

Use the rating system below to track your mood. It will be an excellent reference to look back on! Always be honest, make notes to understand what the three ratings mean to you.

Good ☐ _____

Neutral ☐ _____

Bad ☐ _____

Are you still experiencing cravings at the same points as you did a month ago? Take a look at the triggers you made a note of on Day One to see if they have altered; four weeks is a good length of time to establish a new routine, so with any luck you may notice things have changed during your first month of alcohol-free life. Any cravings for alcohol that you are still experiencing should have dwindled in strength by now.

How have you worked through a craving? Which methods work best in terms of distraction?

"Ignorance is a lot like alcohol; the more you have of it, the less you are able to see its effect on you."

— Jay M. Bylsma

Week 4
Day 6

Today I chose not to drink ☐

Use the rating system below to track your mood. It will be an excellent reference to look back on! Always be honest, make notes to understand what the three ratings mean to you.

Good ☐ _____

Neutral ☐ _____

Bad ☐ _____

If you haven't already done so, make the effort today to arrange a night out. You cannot avoid socialising forever and once you get out there you'll realise that the fear of venturing out sober is much worse than the reality. Make sure that you meet up with friends whose company you enjoy even when not drinking – it sounds obvious but it's amazing how much alcohol covers up, and it really isn't much fun hanging out sober with people who are, when you're not wearing your booze goggles of old, dull as ditch water.

Make a list below of all the friends you truly like, with or without alcohol being a part of the social equation. Prioritise these people when it comes to planning your social calendar.

"Sometimes you have to kind of die inside in order to rise from your own ashes and believe in yourself and love yourself to become a new person."

— Gerard Way (My Chemical Romance)

Lucy's Blog – Happiness, November 25th 2012

Does it sound evangelical to say that I felt complete joy and happiness last night, as I pushed the baby's pram up a steep hill in the driving rain, no hood or hat protecting my head from the downpour and howling gales, and the baby unable to see me or anything else owing to her rain cover being totally misted up with condensation? If I'm honest, I did feel a momentary pang of 'urrghh this is utterly horrible and miserable and I want to be at home in dry clothes, under a blanket in front of the TV.' But only for a minute, and then I reminded myself that I am living and this is what life is about sometimes; taking the dog for a walk in cold, wet weather in the dark.

Everyone tells you that alcohol is a depressant, and you know it's true but somehow it's easy to push that to one side and imagine that your lack of real happiness stems from life just being a bit rubbish.

When you stop drinking alcohol for good, you can experience something akin to an evangelical awakening – moments of happiness that border on delirium, as you realise that you are alive, and lucky for all that you have, and that you've survived stuff and emerged out the other side strong and full of vigour.

I feel joy at seeing the sunrise, listening to the baby wake up, gurgling and burbling to herself in her cot, hearing a song that I love, going for a good run and knowing that I am growing in strength and stamina, having a coffee and a chat with a friend, cooking a new recipe and eating the results.

I am happy nearly every day, at least for most of every day. I do get a bit grumpy or tired, occasionally a little stressed if I'm having a particularly busy and fraught day, but that's just the normal human experience – I would be a robot if I never felt those things. Generally though, I am on an even keel and happiness is the mainstay of my emotions.

I know that's because I don't drink alcohol. It's as simple as that.

Drinking turned me against myself and created an internal battle of depression, anxiety, and self-pity versus normality. Giving it up has allowed the real me to emerge, and the real me is happy and optimistic, calm and centred, full of creativity and determination and passion.

I am eternally grateful that I gave myself the chance to discover who I really am.

Week 4

Day 7

Today I chose not to drink ☐

Use the rating system below to track your mood. It will be an excellent reference to look back on! Always be honest, make notes to understand what the three ratings mean to you.

Good ☐ _____

Neutral ☐ _____

Bad ☐ _____

You have now completed a whole month AF! Give yourself a HUGE pat on the back, take a step back and spend a few moments reflecting on how far you've come. Have a look in the mirror and see how your appearance has altered.

Reward yourself – it's time for your end-of-week treat (remember, whatever you used to spend on booze, spend on something luxurious for YOU).

Write down the 10 best things about being a non-drinker below.

Lucy's Blog – Believe in the Power of Fear, April 28ᵗʰ 2013

I am a big believer in doing what you are scared of. As I watch my 12-month-old crawl around the house with absolutely no sense of fear, it strikes me as obvious that this is how human beings grow and develop awareness of their surroundings – because she isn't scared of attempting the monumental flight of stairs that rise up before her, or knows not to make the descent off the end of the bed head first, Lily gets on with things and learns valuable lessons, such as balance, concentration, focus, and so on. If she was paralysed by fear she would never attempt anything new and would stagnate at the toddler stage of development forever.

As we mature, life delivers a series of (often harsh) lessons that alter the course of our behaviour. We experience something horrible, a memory is created and the next time something similar arises we are naturally cautious. This, together with an increasing sense of mortality, can bring us to a point where we fail to try anything new or remotely scary.

Over the last few years, the events that have frightened me the most are as follows; childbirth, skydiving, flying (particularly taking off and landing), and stopping drinking.

I think you can see where I am going with this – every one of these situations ultimately brought me nothing but immense joy and satisfaction, together with a huge step forward in my personal development. I have only ever known true fear when facing what turned out to be the highlights of my life.

As both my pregnancies approached their natural conclusions I was overwhelmed with a morbid sense of terror regarding the perceived pain and potential medical complications. As the tiny Cessna aircraft climbed to the 10,000 feet drop point, I thought I would literally die with fright – I was utterly petrified and the only reason I actually managed to make the jump was because I was strapped to a man who was clearly going to ignore any protestations on my part about falling two miles to the ground in a matter of minutes.

The biggie for me was facing my fear of sobriety. For reasons which now appear ridiculous, I was scared to death about living my life free from the grip of addiction; terrified of living with clarity and self-awareness, unsure of whom I would be without the stupidity and boring behaviour brought about by my reckless binge drinking. I had a deep sense of foreboding that my life was on the brink of collapse, and that I was facing the rest of my days bored and ascetic, a shadow of my former self.

Fear is there to be faced and overcome. Nowadays whenever something frightens me and my stomach becomes filled with that familiar knot, I remind myself that only good things have ever been born from my fears. I dig deep for courage and just do it.

And with each episode of terror I conquer, my life only gets better.

Week 5

Week 5

Day 1

Today I chose not to drink ☐

Use the rating system below to track your mood. It will be an excellent reference to look back on! Always be honest, make notes to understand what the three ratings mean to you.

Good ☐ _____
_____

Neutral ☐ _____
_____

Bad ☐ _____
_____

A few weeks have passed and complacency may be setting in. Go back to the notes you made in the first week of your six week plan and remind yourself by writing about of bad alcohol has made you feel in the past, and compare it to how much better you feel now. Any notion you have now that things weren't so bad is more than likely the booze talking – if there hadn't been a downside to drinking you wouldn't have bought this book.

Arrive at the decision that you are allergic to ethanol, just as you might be to Brazil nuts or lactose. You have got this far and broken a long-standing habit – the exhaustion that came from drinking, followed by failed attempts to moderate, can only be repeated a few times before it should become blindingly obvious that you and booze will never be great together. Don't fall for the allure of Mr Unsuitable now; remember, this is simply another pathetic attempt at drawing you back in. Stay strong, and keep on being kind to yourself – it will become easier with each passing month.

Week 5
Day 2

Today I chose not to drink ☐

Use the rating system below to track your mood. It will be an excellent reference to look back on! Always be honest, make notes to understand what the three ratings mean to you.

Good ☐ _____
_____

Neutral ☐ _____
_____

Bad ☐ _____
_____

Have you found many new AF drinks yet? Write down some of your favourites, and try this one out for size; it's a great mocktail for those occasions when you crave a drink that's a little bit special ...

Virgin Mojito (serves 2)

Ingredients

Glass full of crushed ice

Half a glass of lemonade or ginger ale

1/4 glass of apple juice

1 tsp brown sugar

8 sprigs of mint

1 lime

Mash the brown sugar with 4 sprigs of the mint. Pour in a little apple juice as you mash. Add the remaining apple juice, lemonade, rest of the mint, and half the lime juice. Stir and pour over the crushed ice. Add the other half of the lime as wedges to serve. This is refreshing and looks very much like the alcoholic variety (good for those who want to blend in with all the boozers).

Week 5
Day 3

Today I chose not to drink ☐

Use the rating system below to track your mood. It will be an excellent reference to look back on! Always be honest, make notes to understand what the three ratings mean to you.

Good ☐ _____
_____

Neutral ☐ _____
_____

Bad ☐ _____
_____

If you are still hearing the whispering of Mr Unsuitable in your ear reassuring you that no harm will come from pouring just one little glass, then take note:

It's time to get tough. Do you want to be a slave to wine o'clock for the rest of your life, or would you love to experience the incredible sense of liberation that comes from being free from your excesses? You will feel empowered if you resist, your self-esteem will begin to grow again and with each occasion you say 'NO!' to alcohol, it will get just that little bit easier.

Use this space to jot down the things you were hoping to get out of becoming AF – have any of them materialised yet?

The Soberistas Tip of the Day:

'I'm running many times a week and meditating every day. This has had the biggest impact in supporting my journey, during times of anxiety and stress, joy and celebration when I would experience a need to change my mood quickly or an automatic thought about having a drink I am learning the art of staying in the moment, grounding myself and being present, not trying to change things but be with the feelings and knowing that feelings aren't permanent. Also thoughts are thoughts, not facts.

Of course life isn't always serene, I still worry and make mistakes, it still rains, people irritate me, and my children drive me nuts, but I don't have wine o'clock anymore.

Finding the Soberistas website on that cold January Sunday offered me a light at the end of the tunnel: I wasn't alone, I could take steps anonymously and build my confidence before outing myself to my nearest and dearest. Giving up alcohol has been the best decision; you really have nothing to lose.'

Lucy's Blog – Goodnight x, May 21st 2013

I've noticed over the last few months how much I love my bedtime. I do have an extremely busy life and am usually exhausted by the time I make my way upstairs to bed and this could be a contributing factor, but since living alcohol-free I have developed a real fondness for hitting the hay.

Night time used to mean drinking; whether at home or out with friends, when the sun went down the wine came out and bedtime was consequently a drunken affair that I barely remembered in the morning (or I would collapse on the settee where I remained comatose and fully clothed until dawn).

At the risk of sounding a little like an old lady, I now find myself enjoying the entire routine of taking my make up off, putting comfortable pyjamas on, and snuggling under the duvet with the low level spotlights creating just enough light for me to read by. When the lights go out I think of all the things I will be doing the next day and feel a sense of happy anticipation for tomorrow, even when there is nothing in particular to be looking forward to. I mentally run over the day I have just had and think of the especially good moments or reflect on the things which perhaps didn't go as I had hoped.

This is most likely a totally normal experience for many people but I'm still enjoying the novelty of it – not waking up with a horrible dry mouth at 5 a.m., no awful arguments or regrettable incidents to agonise over in the dark, early hours when the only company you have is the deeply painful self-hatred that fills every fibre of your being.

I love my cleansers and night moisturisers, my new pyjamas from M&S, the pile of books by my bedside, the feeling of health and freedom of mind, and the knowledge that there will be nothing to be sorry for in the morning. I love feeling sleepy, and that the physical and mental tiredness is because I have worked hard all day and pushed myself to be the best I can be. I love knowing that I won't look like hell in the morning, even if

I'm up during the night with the baby. I love thinking of all the lovely people I have in my life.

I love living and sleeping alcohol-free.

Week 5
Day 4

Today I chose not to drink ☐

Use the rating system below to track your mood. It will be an excellent reference to look back on! Always be honest, make notes to understand what the three ratings mean to you.

Good ☐ _____

Neutral ☐ _____

Bad ☐ _____

Create a cosy bedtime routine for yourself below and make the end of the day a lovely reward for all your efforts to beat the booze. Why not try what Lucy does and stack up a good selection of books by your bedside, treat yourself to a beautiful pair of pyjamas and splash out on some gorgeous skincare products. Remember how you always fell into bed with your make-up on (if you made it that far) and reading was never an option because the words swam before your sozzled eyes? Those days are gone, so be sure to make bedtime extra special – you truly deserve to feel pampered.

"'Why are you drinking?' demanded the little prince.
'So that I may forget,' replied the tippler.
'Forget what?' inquired the little prince, who was already sorry for him.
'Forget that I am ashamed,' the tippler confessed, hanging his head.
'Ashamed of what?' insisted the little prince, who wanted to help him.
'Ashamed of drinking!'"

— Antoine de Saint-Exupéry, *The Little Prince*

Week 5

Day 5

Today I chose not to drink ☐

Use the rating system below to track your mood. It will be an excellent reference to look back on! Always be honest, make notes to understand what the three ratings mean to you.

Good ☐ _____
_____

Neutral ☐ _____
_____

Bad ☐ _____
_____

Now that you have several weeks of AF living behind you, take some time to think about why you used to drink. It is difficult to recognise the reasoning behind our alcohol abuse when our minds are fogged with booze, but with the increased mental clarity that comes with being free from alcohol you should now be able to pinpoint at least a couple of factors that may have contributed to your old drinking habits.

Did you drink to blot out painful feelings? Was it in an effort to overcome social shyness? Are you in an unhappy relationship and you knocked back the wine to try to anaesthetise your daily life?

However painful and however difficult, be honest with yourself and write down over the next couple of pages why you believe you developed such a dependency on alcohol – if you are to successfully conquer this you will need to address whatever underlying issues caused you to turn to the bottle in the first place. It is necessary to carry out a little weeding before new and beautiful flowers can be planted...

Week 5
Day 6

Today I chose not to drink ☐

Use the rating system below to track your mood. It will be an excellent reference to look back on! Always be honest, make notes to understand what the three ratings mean to you.

Good ☐ _____
_____

Neutral ☐ _____
_____

Bad ☐ _____
_____

Use this page to continue with your notes on the reasons behind your alcohol abuse.

Lucy's Blog – Turning the Other Cheek, April 18th 2013

The devil will, I believe, always be within spitting distance of my mind. I'll have days when I ponder the notion that perhaps now, after all this time, I could have just one little drink. That sneaky voice, pervasive and persuasive, will once in a while pop up and proposition me with the questions of 'did you really need to stop for good?' and 'how about you simply exercise some alcohol moderation?' and 'don't you know that time heals all?' I will still, occasionally, feel a tugging on my collar as the demon attempts to lure me back into his den of destruction.

Why can I now resist what I never could during all those drunken years of my past? My sober persistence stems from learning a lesson, accepting the truth and keeping myself firmly on a path that leads in the opposite direction. Being sober and true to myself doesn't mean that I no longer hear the call – it simply means that now I understand the need to ignore it, and that over time I have gradually developed the tools to silence it.

Not drinking alcohol for two years does not eradicate the inability to drink 'sensibly.' Avoiding booze for a sufficient length of time does not magically dissolve the desire to consume the whole bottle just as soon as you pop the cork and swallow your first mouthful. But what time without alcohol does provide is enough self-awareness to allow you to recognise your weak spots, your triggers, and your instincts.

Living alcohol-free allows you to develop the knowledge that your brain operates on two levels; this is commonly referred to as being ruled by your head or your heart, or having your angel on one shoulder and the devil on the other. Given enough time without alcohol sullying your ability to think clearly, it becomes second nature to spot which is the 'bad brain' talking and which is you.

A little like being a child and having a naughty friend who coerces you into causing trouble with them, and a good, loyal friend who respects you and regards your feelings above their own, understanding which of your two brains to listen to means arriving at the realisation of what's right for you, and what works best in your happy life.

So when you hear that little voice whispering sweet nothings in your ear and attempting to draw you back to where you ran so desperately from once upon a time, try and regard it as the bad friend – turn the other cheek and seek out what's right. YOU will thank you for your strength in the morning.

Week 5

Day 7

Today I chose not to drink ☐

Use the rating system below to track your mood. It will be an excellent reference to look back on! Always be honest, make notes to understand what the three ratings mean to you.

Good ☐ _____

Neutral ☐ _____

Bad ☐ _____

Well done – you have reached the end of a difficult week. While there are many obvious bonuses to an alcohol-free life (more energy, an even mood leading to more settled relationships, possible weight loss, more spare time, better self-esteem, and so on), you are still working through long-established habits and the associated cravings.

As the initial impetus to stop drinking alcohol diminishes over time, so the rose-tinted glasses will come out, painting a beautifully edited picture of all the good times you shared with your old flame Mr Unsuitable.

It takes much inner strength to ignore these tempting thoughts, and it takes a while for such mental teasing to die down. Write about how you overcame these thoughts today, then congratulate yourself, buy something nice, and relax ... you've almost completed your six week plan!

"When you quit drinking you stop waiting."

— Caroline Knapp

Week 6

Week 6
Day 1

Today I chose not to drink ☐

Use the rating system below to track your mood. It will be an excellent reference to look back on! Always be honest, make notes to understand what the three ratings mean to you.

Good ☐ _____

Neutral ☐ _____

Bad ☐ _____

You may discover that now you've begun the final week of your six week plan, the Wine Witch has begun to whisper little suggestions in your ear about celebrating your month and a half of sobriety by downing a few glasses of the old poison. Remind yourself that you are still operating under the influence of well-established boozy habits, and it will take a while for your brain to rewire itself.

If you give into temptation you would not be treating yourself but undoing all the hard work you have put in over the last few weeks – remember that in order to allow yourself room to change you must learn to say no to the addictive voice in your head. This time you are looking for a long term strategy, and while you have begun the job of reconfiguring your mental processes, you should now harness all your inner strength in order to finish the job properly.

Have you fantasised about celebrating your sober success to date with a bottle of fizz? Remember the 'Play the Movie to the End' trick and jot down below how you foresee things turning out, should you cave in (and be honest!):

Some people can drink alcohol moderately and manage to maintain a happy, balanced life.

Some people cannot.

Alcohol can make you feel happy, sexy, confident, and full of *joie de vivre*.

Alcohol can make you feel desperately unhappy, full of self-hatred, anxious, and sick.

Drinking is a social event, a 'thing' that seems to be all around us.

Being teetotal can, on occasion, make you feel left out.

Nobody can make you stop drinking, so if you choose, you can continue to drink until you die.

Nobody can make you continue to drink, so if you choose, you never have to drink alcohol again.

Some people can take or leave alcohol.

Some people can't seem to stop drinking once they begin.

Some people want to reach self-fulfilment.

Some people are happy to drift along as they are.

Alcohol is marketed in a way which can make it appear to be sophisticated and cool.

Alcohol is the root cause of thousands of deaths every year.

Alcohol can negatively skew your vision of your world.

You possess the ability to choose what works best for you in your life.

You are the master of your own destiny.

Week 6
Day 2

Today I chose not to drink ☐

Use the rating system below to track your mood. It will be an excellent reference to look back on! Always be honest, make notes to understand what the three ratings mean to you.

Good ☐ _____
_____

Neutral ☐ _____
_____

Bad ☐ _____
_____

Throughout the last few sober weeks all sorts of suggestions and ideas may have popped into your mind. Once the booze fog lifts it can feel as though the brain has gone into overdrive. You may have taken stock of your life and come up with some pretty radical ideas as to how you would like your future to unfold. As your headspace fills up with all these extra thoughts it can sometimes feel a little overwhelming – write down here some of the ideas you have pondered over these last few weeks, and look closely at the ones you would like to put into action. Perhaps now would be a good time to engage in further investigations with regards to getting the ball rolling with some aspects of your new life.

"Who in the world am I? Ah, that's the great puzzle."

— Lewis Carroll, *Alice in Wonderland*

Week 6

Day 3

Today I chose not to drink ☐

Use the rating system below to track your mood. It will be an excellent reference to look back on! Always be honest, make notes to understand what the three ratings mean to you.

Good ☐ _____
_____

Neutral ☐ _____
_____

Bad ☐ _____
_____

By now you should have thrown out some of your internal baggage, whether this has been through talking with friends and family, or simply thinking things through with the increased clarity that AF living offers. While in the middle of it, this process can be incredibly painful but it is absolutely necessary if you are to move on positively from your alcohol dependency. Once things are out in the open they no longer fester internally, freeing you up to make room for happiness again.

Write down the main issues which you feel you have begun to work through during the last six weeks; how do you feel about them now? Do you feel any lighter emotionally?

Week 6
Day 4

Today I chose not to drink ☐

Use the rating system below to track your mood. It will be an excellent reference to look back on! Always be honest, make notes to understand what the three ratings mean to you.

Good ☐ _____
_____

Neutral ☐ _____
_____

Bad ☐ _____
_____

Do some calculations this week on finances. Do not sweep anything under the booze carpet. How much you have saved, not only on home drinking, but in all the other associated ways we manage to haemorrhage money when we drink frequently and heavily; it might just surprise you to see how much you have NOT spent on alcohol over the last six weeks.

If you thought a designer handbag was expensive check out your annual drip feed of wine bottles. A £6 bottle of wine per day adds up to well over £2000 a year, and that's not including all those little drunken add-ons we have all been guilty of frittering our money on when under the influence … (pizza, fags, a weekend away on Lastminute.com; these ring any bells?!)What could you spend £2000 on in a year's time? Think about opening a savings account purely for your booze money and watch the balance build up over the next 12 months. Jot down some more ideas below on how you could put that cash to good use:

"If you ever know a woman who tries to drown her sorrows, kindly inform her sorrows know how to swim."

— Pittacus Lore, *The Power of Six*

Week 6
Day 5

Today I chose not to drink ☐

Use the rating system below to track your mood. It will be an excellent reference to look back on! Always be honest, make notes to understand what the three ratings mean to you.

Good ☐ _____

Neutral ☐ _____

Bad ☐ _____

Although getting rid of Mr Unsuitable is all about you and restoring your self-esteem, you will probably have noticed by now some pleasing side effects on those around you stemming from your decision to cut out alcohol.

As your mood levels out and the cravings become more manageable, thus reducing any tension and stress, your family and friends will more than likely have begun to respond to you in a more positive manner. Have you noticed that you are more patient and understanding with your loved ones? Has there been a particular instance when you felt that by being sober you were able to be a better mum, friend, or partner?

Make a note here of how being sober has helped improve your close relationships:

Week 6

Day 6

Today I chose not to drink ☐

Use the rating system below to track your mood. It will be an excellent reference to look back on! Always be honest, make notes to understand what the three ratings mean to you.

Good ☐ _____
                _____

Neutral ☐ _____
                  _____

Bad ☐ _____
             _____

Take a few moments to reflect on how you have changed during the course of the last six weeks; have you discovered that you enjoy a hobby or fitness activity which was something you would never have dreamt of doing once upon a drunken time? Do you feel better physically, and have you seen any improvements in your appearance? How is your mental state – have you suffered from depression or anxiety during the last few weeks or has your mood lifted?

Any positive results that have occurred as a result of eliminating alcohol from your life should be celebrated – it is no coincidence that life tends to get easier when you put down the bottle, so be sure to acknowledge all the benefits with the recognition that they have occurred as a direct result of you making the brilliant decision to NOT DRINK ALCOHOL!

By noticing the positive effects of alcohol-free living, and by fully appreciating why these things have begun to take shape, you are creating a stock of helpful reasoning to be drawn on next time you feel the slightest temptation to reach for the bottle. Make sure you write the most positive effects that you've noticed below.

Week 6

Day 7

Today I chose not to drink ☐

Use the rating system below to track your mood. It will be an excellent reference to look back on! Always be honest, make notes to understand what the three ratings mean to you.

Good ☐ _____
_____

Neutral ☐ _____
_____

Bad ☐ _____
_____

We hope that you are feeling immensely proud of your accomplishments today; not only have you successfully completed six weeks of sober living, but hopefully you have worked through some longstanding and difficult issues which will help make you more aware of the reasons why you began to drink so heavily in the first instance.

By recording your feelings as you have progressed through the six weeks you have created a highly valuable and personal guide to beating your alcohol dependency for good. Not only does it help to write down your thoughts as a way of processing them, but by keeping a diary you now have something to return to time and time again should you ever experience days when Mr Unsuitable begins to creep back into your thoughts.

Hopefully as time goes by this will happen less and less, but whenever that voice pops up you will be better equipped to deal with it.

Take another photo of yourself and compare it to the one you took before you started Your 6 Week Plan. The extent of the results could well be surprising, with lost weight, clearer skin, and brighter eyes. Isn't this the you that you want to see for good?

Well done for making it through Your 6 Week Plan; write down one sentence below that sums up your feelings on your massive achievement:

"I would not put a thief in my mouth to steal my brains."

— William Shakespeare, *Othello*

I've been picking up on stories across the media and in random conversations, that we non-drinkers have been labelled by some as the 'New Puritans.' This label suggests that we have a rather holier-than-thou attitude, as if we are in some way superior and a bit boring; religious nuts, health freaks, or incredibly dull.

It's true that we don't get roaring drunk anymore or even giddy with the assistance of alcohol. We are giddy enough without it. It's also true that we are sharp, savvy, and on time, with a straightforward perspective on how life is. We don't pull sickies, nor do we have lost days or weekends. There are no blackouts, no embarrassing and shameful covering up to deal with, there is no waking up in strange places with a mouth that feels like the inside of Gandhi's flip-flop.

Women who get their control and lives back through becoming AF often have a bucket list longer than their arm because they have a lot of catching up to do and are excited about life again.

Do any of us non-drinkers become puritanical preachers? Most I know are really happy with their new lifestyle of clarity but not at all keen to thrust it on anyone else unless they really want to follow suit – and then it is with gentleness and empathy.

Pub culture from the olden days seems so romantic and jolly, and if pubs were still like that, it would be wonderful for the community, especially in rural areas. No wide-screen TVs' showing football, or loud music, just adult conversation with a smattering of gossip.

By and large, the non-drinkers I know really don't judge anyone, for anything. So why is it, when women like us who have at last got our lives under control, looking and feeling great are judged as boring puritans by drinkers? We faced stigma as drunks, and still face it sober.

There is so much defensiveness and denial associated with

136

booze, and this really comes across in the comments following online newspaper articles about heavy drinkers. People pile in with the usual tirades about how it's their life and they'll live it their way. Well good for them – all I hope for is that it never descends into the chaos that ours did as a result of alcohol.

If sobriety is becoming more fashionable then I am delighted. Any woman in control of her life is a force to be reckoned with, but perhaps that might just be frightening to some people. In our less-than-boring circles, we are very grateful to be a part of the new wave – it's golden, and you know what? It's catching on. Welcome to the Sober Revolution!

CONGRATULATIONS – YOU MADE IT!

Your Six Week Plan is a reminder of where you once were, and, more importantly, how far you have come. Treasure it, for it will be a vital element of your armoury should you experience any waves of boozy temptation in the future.

"If you want to understand the causes that existed in the past, look at the results as they are manifested in the present. And if you want to understand what results will be manifested in the future, look at the causes that exist in the present." – Buddhist Quote

After passing their driving test many people are under the impression that they are suddenly the world's best driver. They drive too fast without any comprehension of the responsibility that has been granted to them as a result of being freed of their learner plates, and it often takes many years before they sufficiently mature behind the wheel to recognise that, actually, the learning only just begins at the test-passing stage; it is the years of driving independently, making choices alone without an instructor guiding you along, perhaps having the odd bump or more serious accident, that build up a true ability to drive.

Now that you have successfully completed *Your Six Week*

Plan, it would be wise to consider yourself to be at the same stage as the driver who has just passed her test; you've got the tools, you've had the guidance, now it's time to embark on a steady learning curve through day-to-day life.

Your Six Week Plan gives you the opportunity to utilise a lasting account of your personal journey for sober success. In addition to the notes you have collated throughout the last few weeks, you can also log on to Soberistas.com for a solid support resource.

Remember that, rather than drinking because of each and every problem life throws at you, you should now try to find the strength to face them head on. You only have to take the first step into clear and reasoned confrontation – after that the rest will be doable. Plan it, consider it, and deal with it. Patience and wisdom walk hand in hand, and both are very cool. Prove to yourself and others that you are a woman of substance and self-worth. Being in control of your life and fulfilling your potential is both sexy and savvy – make your sobriety work in the most positive way for you.

With regards to the objectives of your new alcohol-free life, the most important is to secure your emotional wellbeing. Linked to this is the ability to ensure your optimum health and happiness in order for you to remain a pivotal component of your family. Another is to demonstrate both to you and those around you that discovering true contentment and having fun are not about getting hammered but about being someone who makes a lasting impression for all the best reasons, rather than the embarrassing and regrettable ones. You will never have looked or felt better.

Any lingering self-doubts can finally, with a clear head, be tackled – flaws can be embraced and converted to personal strengths. With the clarity you will now have, as well as the extra energy, time and money, full potential can and should be realised. No more procrastination, no more fear.

Remember to avoid being either smug or evangelical; the Sober Revolution is about being chic and subtle. No holier than thou attitudes for us, we exude both compassion and kindness, but most importantly, power. It's a heady mix. Just let your actions speak for themselves, and they will say more than enough.

Compendium

Good Health & the Imaginary Cashmere Blanket

As soon as you have made the choice to quit drinking alcohol you should focus on taking good care of yourself, especially for the initial few weeks – wrap yourself in an imaginary cashmere blanket and make it your priority to meet the needs of both body and mind.

Alcohol abuse and a disregard for one's physical and mental wellbeing quite often go hand in hand, therefore becoming AF means learning how to be kind to yourself – perhaps for the first time in your adult life. Key to this self-love is getting into the habit of providing your body with excellent nutrition to repair some of the physical damage caused by excessive alcohol consumption, and to boost your mental state in order to maximise your chance at sober success.

You may not feel ready to go all out on a domestic goddess vibe and this isn't necessary unless you really feel the urge. Keeping it simple is sometimes the best option as complicated preparation of fancy meals is, for many, a trigger for pouring a large glass of vino – if this sounds like you then simplicity really should you be your goal, for the time being at least.

Vitamin B1 – Facts and Foods

It is widely acknowledged that chronic abuse of alcohol can result in a deficiency in thiamine (also known as vitamin B1). A lack of vitamin B1 negatively affects the brain in a number of ways, in particular causing a wide range of deficits in cognition, behaviour patterns, and motor coordination. As insurance, it is wise to take a vitamin B complex supplement daily, but read on for some easy and delicious meal ideas which are packed full of thiamine.

There is an abundance of foods which are simple to prepare and full of vitamin B1. Remember that most of us think in pictures rather than words and therefore we need to change our mental image of reward from a glass of wine, to nutritious food and health-giving treats. Just as we have, on many past occasions, conjured up a fantasy picture of how glamorous we look with a glass of our favourite tipple to hand, now is the time to start working on a new, chic visual which sees you brimming with natural health and confidence, fully in control of your life and enjoying supplying your body with the nutrients it deserves.

Bear in mind, too, now that you aren't breaking the bank with an unaffordable alcohol habit, you might have some surplus cash which can be spent more wisely on good quality ingredients for rustling up a range of delicious and nutritious meals.

Vitamin B1-Rich Meal Ideas

Love it or hate it, Marmite is stuffed full of vitamin B – quick and easy for use as a spread, or add a spoonful into baked beans and serve with granary toast.

Sesame seeds, flaxseeds, and sunflower seeds are all full of this much-needed vitamin. Make a mixture of these seeds and store in a couple of containers – keep one handy for snacking in the kitchen and one in the car too for when hunger strikes while on the move. Hummus with pitta bread is excellent for staving off a tummy rumble too, and if you buy the lower fat variety it's not that heavy on the calories either.

For a more substantial hit of vitamin B1, pork chops are ideal. Simple to cook, make sure you buy good organic pork if you can afford it. Try serving with a mustard and apple sauce mixed with crème fraiche, and a root vegetable mash – 30 minutes start to finish. Simple!

If you are a fish fan, both salmon and tuna are B1 rich. Straightforward and quick to prepare – accompany either with broccoli, spring onions and ginger. These health-giving fish meals will provide you with a real boost.

Soups are a fabulous way to pack a whole host of nutritious foods into a speedy and scrumptious meal; you can make one when you are in the mood or have some spare time (there should be much more of that now you've ditched the booze!) – make more than one portion and refrigerate or freeze for future use. On a chilly evening, potato, spinach and leek soup is glorious and warming; for a lighter dish, try making chicken and sweetcorn soup (sweetcorn is another source of vitamin B1).

Potato, Spinach, & Leek Soup

Ingredients

Knob of butter

2 cloves of garlic

1 onion

2 leeks, washed and finely sliced

250g fresh spinach

Handful thyme leaves

250g of potatoes, washed and diced

1 litre vegetable stock

155g mascarpone cheese

Melt a knob of butter in a large pan and gently fry the garlic, an onion, the leeks, spinach, thyme and potatoes. After a few minutes add the vegetable stock, bring to the boil and simmer for half an hour – make sure the potatoes are tender. Take off the heat and whizz with a handheld blender. Stir through the mascarpone cheese and season to taste with salt and black pepper. Serve with crusty bread.

Chicken & Sweetcorn Soup

Ingredients

150g chicken breast

1 clove of garlic

1cm piece of fresh ginger, grated

800ml chicken stock

1 tbsp cornflour

150g sweetcorn (frozen or tinned)

Handful spring onions, roughly chopped

Splash soy sauce

In a large pan, fry (in a tablespoon of vegetable oil) the chicken, garlic, and ginger. Thicken the chicken stock with the cornflour and add to the chicken with the sweetcorn. Bring to the boil and simmer for about ten minutes. Stir in the spring onions and splash of soy sauce before serving.

Other Vitamins and Supplements

Excessive alcohol consumption can also result in a depletion of vitamin C, otherwise known as ascorbic acid. If you have ever noticed unexplained bruising on your body, a deficiency in this vitamin may be the reason – vitamin C is required for the body's production of collagen which is necessary for connective tissue maintenance and repair.

A severe deficiency of vitamin C is known as scurvy, commonly suffered by sailors during the 18th century. The symptoms of scurvy include the deterioration of blood vessels, bleeding gums, loss of hair, nails and teeth, and in the most serious cases, heart failure. A mild case of vitamin C can lead to frequent bruising, a weakened immune system, and joint pain.

Some fantastic foods to consume for restoring the body's

vitamin C levels are red and green chilli peppers, dark green leafy vegetables (such as curly kale), broccoli, guavas, kiwis, papayas, strawberries, and oranges. Try making a delicious fruit salad that utilises some or all of the fruits listed here.

The Liver

Of all the organs that take a battering from heavy boozing, the liver suffers the most. Luckily, cell regeneration of the liver is incredibly fast with each single cell being replaced approximately every forty days. Below is a list of the symptoms of a sluggish liver – see if any of them are familiar to you:

§   Tiredness, fatigue

§   Headaches

§   Bad breath

§   Allergies and food intolerance

§   Problem skin

§   Weight gain

§   Anxiety/depression

§   Impaired libido

§   PMS

§   Nausea

§   Vomiting

§   Abdominal pain

§   Jaundice

§   Darkened urine

For foods which encourage liver regeneration you need to think green, fresh, and un-processed.

Green leafy vegetables that are rich in iron and magnesium, and those that contain high levels of chlorophyll, are all very efficient liver cleansers. Chlorophyll-rich foods include, of course, green leafy vegetables of all kinds, green olives, romaine lettuce, sea vegetables, broccoli, green peas, leeks, bell peppers, and wheatgrass juice. Spinach is also an excellent source of chlorophyll.

Sulphur is another vital mineral, important in the protection of your body from the toxins and heavy metals found in our environment. It has been widely acknowledged for its healing properties for thousands of years.

Up your intake of sulphur by eating foods which include nuts, cabbage, Brussels sprouts, onions, leek, garlic, watercress, kelp, grape juice, coconut milk and avocado.

Cranberry is your friend now and here's a really easy tonic to make up in a 2 litre jug; one part unsweetened cranberry juice to 8 parts filtered water. Fill up a juice bottle to take to work or when you are out and about. Ideally you should be drinking at least this amount a day for the first 10 days as you need to hydrate. Your skin will also thank you for it.

NB Reserve plenty of space in your schedule for 'you time' now that the focus is off the wine aisle. When food shopping, take a few moments to look and feel fresh produce before it goes into the basket or trolley – be patient and mindful of what you will be putting into your body. After sustained alcohol abuse it is important to repair some of the damage – your body is the only one you've got, so start to look after it now with care and gentleness.

More AF Drinks Ideas

Earlier in the plan we discussed the acronym HALT – wherever possible try to avoid becoming hungry, angry, lonely, and/or tired. Be sure to allow yourself as much rest as possible in the first few weeks of sobriety as your body begins to recover from the excess alcohol. With regards to ensuring that your body never becomes hungry, a good stock of smoothie ingredients is worth maintaining in your kitchen, as a smoothie is a fast and nutritious way to fill up quickly.

Make sure you keep plenty of milk, yoghurt, and apple juice in the fridge as these can form the basis of a variety of smoothie recipes. In addition, go mad in the fruit aisle when you do the shopping! Melons, strawberries, cherries, bananas, blueberries, blackberries, and mango are great fresh options for fruit but don't forget that dried fruit such as apricots and dates also work well, as do tinned and frozen varieties of a number of different fruits.

Other than that just invest in a decent blender, ensuring it is one which is relatively easy to clean so that the washing up afterwards doesn't put you off using it! For the following smoothie recipes simply throw the ingredients into a blender (chop the fruit beforehand) and blend until smooth.

Banana & Melon Smoothie

1 banana

½ cantaloupe melon

2 strawberries

A cup of ice cubes

200 g of coconut yogurt

Apricot & Banana Smoothie

1 banana

Handful of dried apricots

Sprinkling of omega 3-rich seed mix (from health stores and most large supermarkets)

200 g of plain yoghurt

100 ml apple juice

Lassis

A lassi is a yoghurt-based drink which originates from the Punjab region of India. Traditional lassi are savoury, often flavoured with cumin. However, sweet lassis have seen a recent surge in popularity in Western cultures, with mango lassi being particularly in favour. Lassis are incredibly malleable in terms of ingredients – basically, other than the yoghurt (and there is room for choice there too as you can opt for fat-free, Greek, or plain natural – whatever floats your boat! – you are free to stick in whatever takes your fancy. However, here are a few tips that you may wish to follow:

- Consume soon after making – lassis don't keep terribly well.

- If you have a sweet tooth then consider using alternative sweeteners to plain old sugar – honey or maple syrup both work well. Seasonal fruit which is ripe and ready-to-eat is naturally sweeter than its unripe or out-of-season counterpart so choose wisely when shopping for produce.

- You can use ice, although in our opinion, lassis are best made without – if you do decide to go down the iceless route, ensure that the yoghurt and other ingredients are nicely chilled prior to blending.

Here are a few of our favourite lassi recipes, all of which serve 2 (simply throw ingredients into a blender and blend until smooth):

Mango Lassi

150ml single cream

200ml full-fat milk

200ml plain yoghurt

400 g mango chunks (roughly the flesh of 2 large mangoes)

2 dollops of honey

Optional extra – smashed pistachios to garnish

Apple & Blueberry Lassi

400 ml plain yoghurt

150 ml full fat milk

50 ml apple juice

2 dessert apples, cored and cut into chunks

200 g blueberries

2 dollops of honey

Coconut & Honey Lassi

1 480 ml tin of coconut water

1 480 ml tin of low fat coconut milk

150 ml plain yoghurt

2 tbsps desiccated coconut

2 dollops of manuka honey

1/4 tsp cinnamon

1/8 tsp nutmeg

Optional extra – flaked coconut for garnish

If you are looking for a delicious alternative to your old alcoholic beverage of choice, you may wish to find something that is simple to make, with ingredients that are cheap and easy to obtain. Especially in the first few days and weeks of sobriety you should aim to find a drink that has all the ready availability of, say, wine or beer. If a replacement involves too much faff then you may be dissuaded from making it, finding it all too easy to fall back into old habits.

With this in mind, see below for a round-up of some really

quick and easy drinks ideas that you can knock up in a couple of minutes:

- Elderflower cordial with sparkling water and ice

- Ginger cordial, sparkling water and ice – with a twist of fresh lemon juice, a grating of fresh ginger and a sprig of mint to garnish

- Ginger beer over ice

- Hot chocolate (made as instructed on packet) with a spoonful of Nutella and a dollop of whipped cream – for a special treat on a cold night!

- Pineapple juice mixed with lemonade, served over ice

- (One to make in advance) – Fill a large container (one with a lid) with cold water and add 6 – 8 herbal tea bags (fruity flavours work best), leaving the strings hanging over the edge. Trap the strings with the lid and close tight. Place in the fridge overnight. Remove the teabags before serving in tall glasses with ice and a sprig of fresh mint to garnish.

- As above but use regular teabags instead; serve with a slice of fresh lemon to garnish.

- Peach Bel-tea-ni; mix peach ice tea with peach juice (available in Tesco & Waitrose), add a few mint

leaves and a cup full of ice. Top up with soda water
or lemonade.

- Strawberry Juice (use Pago Juices available from
Amazon if you can't find this anywhere else) topped
up with lemonade. Add frozen strawberries instead
of ice.

Disclaimer

For many people, there is no substitute for professional therapy with a counsellor who specialises in alcohol addiction. This book is not a replacement for this, nor any other type of recognised alcohol addiction support/therapy, but an additional support resource that may complement your other endeavours to control your consumption of alcohol. If you are struggling with an alcohol dependency or are at all worried about your alcohol consumption, please discuss with your GP in the first instance.

For contact details of alcohol support groups, please visit the Soberistas website.

Join The Sober Revolution
and call time on wine o'clock

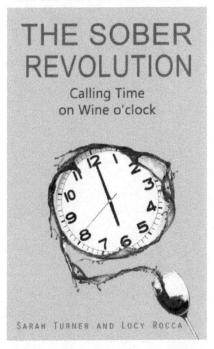

The Sober Revolution looks at women and their relationships
with alcohol, exploring the myths behind this socially
acceptable yet often destructive habit. Rather than continuing
the sad spiral into addiction it helps women regain control of
their drinking and live happier, healthier lives.

Sarah Turner, cognitive behavioural therapist and addictions
counsellor, and Lucy Rocca, founder of Soberistas.com,
the popular social networking site for women who have
successfully kicked the booze or would like to, give an insight
into ways to find a route out of the world of wine.